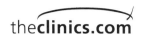

CLINICS IN PODIATRIC MEDICINE AND SURGERY OF NORTH AMERICA

Diagnosis and Treatment of Peripheral Nerve Entrapments and Neuropathy

GUEST EDITOR
Babak Baravarian, DPM

CONSULTING EDITOR
Vincent J. Mandracchia, DPM, MS

July 2006 • Volume 23 • Number 3

SAUNDERS

An Imprint of Elsevier, Inc.
PHILADELPHIA   LONDON   TORONTO   MONTREAL   SYDNEY   TOKYO

W.B. SAUNDERS COMPANY
A Division of Elsevier Inc.

1600 John F. Kennedy Bldv., Suite 1800, Philadelphia, PA 19103-2899

http://www.theclinics.com

CLINICS IN PODIATRIC MEDICINE   Volume 23, Number
AND SURGERY   ISSN 0891-842
July 2006   ISBN 1-4160-3880-
Editor: Alexandra Gavenda

The ideas and opinion expressed in *Clinics in Podiatric Medicine and Surgery* do not necessarily reflect thos of the Publisher. The Publisher does not assume any responsibility for any injury and/or damage to per sons or property arising out of or related to any use of the material contained in this periodical. The reade is advised to check the appropriate medical literature and the product information currently provided b the manufacturer of each drug to be administered to verify the dosage, the method and duration of admin istration, or contraindications. It is the responsibility of the treating physician or other health care profes sional, relying on independent experience and knowledge of the patient, to determine drug dosages an the best treatment for the patient. Mention of any product in this issue should not be construed as endorse ment by the contributors, editors, or the Publisher of the product of manufacturers' claims.

Reprints. For copies of 100 or more of articles in this publication, please contact the Commercial Reprint Department, Elsevier Inc., 360 Park Avenue South, New York, New York 10010-1710 Tel.: (212) 633-3813 Fax: (212) 462-1935, e-mail: reprints@elsevier.com

Clinics in Podiatric Medicine and Surgery (ISSN 0891-8422) is published quarterly by Elsevier Inc., 360 Par Avenue South, New York, NY 10010-1710. Months of publication are January, April, July, and Octobe Business and Editorial Offices: 1600 John F. Kennedy Blvd., Suite 1800, Philadelphia, PA 191023-2899. Cus tomer Service Office: 6277 Sea Harbor Drive, Orlando, FL 32887-4800. Periodicals postage paid at Nev York, NY, and additional mailing offices. Subscription prices are $175.00 per year for US individual $280.00 per year for US institutions, $90.00 per year for US students and residents, $210.00 per year fo Canadian individuals, $340.00 for Canadian institutions, $235.00 for international individuals, $340.0(per year for international institutions and $120.00 per year for Canadian and foreign students/resident To receive student/resident rate, orders must be accompanied by name of affiliated institution, date o term, and the *signature* of program/residency coordinator on institution letterhead. Orders will be bille at individual rate until proof of status is received. Foreign air speed delivery is included in all *Clinics* sub scription prices. All prices are subject to change without notice. POSTMASTER: Send address changes t(*Clinics in Podiatric Medicine and Surgery,* Elsevier Periodicals Customer Service, 6277 Sea Harbor Drive, Or lando, FL 32887-4800. **Customer Service: 1-800-654-2452 (US). From outside of the US, call 1-407-345 1000.**

Clinics in Podiatric Medicine and Surgery is covered in *Index Medicus* and *EMBASE/Excerpta Medica.*

Printed in the United States of America.

CONSULTING EDITOR

VINCENT J. MANDRACCHIA, DPM, MS, Section Chief, Podiatric Surgery, Department of Surgery, Broadlawns Medical Center; Clinical Professor, Department of Podiatric Medicine and Surgery, College of Podiatric Medicine and Surgery, Des Moines University–Osteopathic Medicine Center, Des Moines, Iowa

GUEST EDITOR

BABAK BARAVARIAN, DPM, Assistant Clinical Professor, UCLA School of Medicine, Los Angeles, California; Chief of Foot and Ankle Surgery, Santa Monica/UCLA Medical Center, Santa Monica, California; Director, Foot and Ankle Institute Network, Los Angeles, California

CONTRIBUTORS

BABAK BARAVARIAN, DPM, Assistant Clinical Professor, UCLA School of Medicine, Los Angeles, California; Chief of Foot and Ankle Surgery, Santa Monica/UCLA Medical Center, Santa Monica, California; Director, Foot and Ankle Institute Health Network, Los Angeles, California

STEPHEN L. BARRETT, DPM, MBA, FACFAS, CWS, Associate Professor, Midwestern University, College of Health Sciences, Arizona Podiatric Medicine Program, Glendale, Arizona

BRADLEY D. BEASLEY, DPM, AACFAS, Metro Tulsa Foot and Ankle Specialists, Broken Arrow, Oklahoma

TAMARA J. BOND, PT, Director of Physical Therapy Services, Foot and Ankle Institute of Santa Monica, Santa Monica, California

WILLIAM G. BUXTON, MD, Assistant Clinical Professor of Neurology, David Geffen School of Medicine at UCLA, Los Angeles, California; UCLA-Santa Monica Neurologic Associates, Santa Monica, California; California Subspecialty Certification in Clinical Neurophysiology

ANNE T. CHRISTOPHER, MD, FAAPMR, Pain Evaluation and Treatment Center, Tulsa, Oklahoma

A. LEE DELLON, MD, Professor of Plastic Surgery and Neurosurgery, Johns Hopkins University, Baltimore, Maryland; Clinical Professor of Plastic Surgery, Neurosurgery, and Anatomy, University of Arizona, Tucson, Arizona; Director of the Dellon Institutes for Peripheral Nerve, Baltimore, Maryland, Boston, Massachusetts, and Tucson, Arizona

LAWRENCE A. DI DOMENICO, DPM, FACFAS, Adjunct Professor, Ohio College of Podiatric Medicine, Department of Surgery, Northside Medical Center, Youngstown, Ohio

JUSTIN E. DOMINICK, MD, Assistant Clinical Professor of Neurology, David Geffen School of Medicine at UCLA, Los Angeles, California; UCLA-Santa Monica Neurologic Associates, Santa Monica; California Diplomate, American Board of Electrodiagnostic Medicine

DAVID A. FRANCIS, DPM, FACFAS, Green Country Podiatry Center, Tulsa, Oklahoma

JUSTIN FRANSON, DPM, Clinical Instructor, UCLA School of Medicine, Los Angeles, California; Instructor, Veterans Hospital, Los Angeles, California; Director, Foot and Ankle Institute of Valencia, Valencia, California

CHRISTOPHER HELLER, JR, BS, University of Arizona, College of Medicine, Tucson, Arizona

JIM LUNDY, DPT, CSCS, Director of Physical Therapy Services, Athletic Physical Therapy, Los Angeles, California

CHRISTOPHER T. MALONEY, JR, MD, Clinical Assistant Professor of Surgery and Neurosurgery, Department of Surgery, University of Arizona, Tucson, Arizona

ERIC B. MASTERNICK, DPM, AAFCAS, Private Practice, Youngstown, Ohio

JOSHUA R. OLSON, BS, Medical Student, University of Arizona, College of Medicine, Tucson, Arizona

GEDGE D. ROSSON, MD, Assistant Professor, Division of Plastic, Reconstructive, and Maxillofacial Surgery, Johns Hopkins University School of Medicine, Baltimore, Maryland; The Dellon Institutes for Peripheral Nerve Surgery, Baltimore, Maryland

DAVID SOOMEKH, DPM, The Foot and Ankle Institute of Santa Monica, Santa Monica, California; Clinical Instructor, UCLA Medical Center, Santa Monica, California

CONTENTS

> Currently there is unprecedented interest in research, writing, and clinical experience related to lower extremity peripheral nerve surgery. Its time is here, now. Application of the concepts for diagnosis and treatment of nerve compression, painful neuroma, and neuropathy has been a direct extension from the upper extremity to the lower extremity. By the end of 2005, there were more than a dozen studies demonstrating that the basic neuropathy causes metabolic changes that render the peripheral nerve susceptible to chronic nerve compressions. My hypothesis continues to assert that surgical decompression of known sites of compression can relieve symptoms of neuropathy that are caused by superimposed nerve compressions.

> There are many types of peripheral nerve disorders that lead to peripheral neuropathy. Symptoms associated with peripheral neuropathy lack consistent, easy to treat qualities, and provide a

constant challenge for physicians who encounter the sequelae of neuropathy. This review discusses medications, nutritional supplements, and topical and physical modalities that are effective in treating neuropathy associated with diabetes.

Electrodiagnostic testing (EDX), the combination of electromyography and nerve conduction studies, is a useful extension of the physical exam. In the proper clinical context, it can help distinguish between the various nerve processes that may contribute to foot pain. This article discusses those processes, their clinical presentation, and the relative usefulness of EDX for each.

The diagnosis and treatment of peripheral neuropathy from any cause has come to the forefront of the research community in the past few years. Both past and new diagnostic and treatment options have been and are being studied to better understand and properly treat this debilitating and sometimes devastating disease. One such advancement is the clinical use of quantitative sensory testing. To identify etiology of the neuropathy early, the testing instrument would need to identify changes throughout the course of the disease, have a normative database, and show a clear distinction between the absence or presence of disease. The pressure specified sensory device (PSSD) was developed in 1992 to painlessly investigate the cutaneous pressure thresholds quantitatively and accurately.

For years, patients who were treated successfully with carpal tunnel release were told there was nothing that could be done about their lower extremity symptoms. Now that lower extremity nerve decompression has been accepted as an option to treat appropriate patients, the authors looked for correlations between a successful outcome with carpal tunnel syndrome and its predictive value of success for lower extremity nerve decompression. Data from a recent study demonstrate that a good result from upper extremity peripheral nerve surgery predicts the outcome for lower extremity peripheral nerve surgery in 88% of patients, and is, therefore, information valuable for prognosis and clinical decision-making.

FORTHCOMING ISSUES

RECENT ISSUES

THE CLINICS ARE NOW AVAILABLE ONLINE!

http://www.theclinics.com

ELSEVIER
SAUNDERS

Clin Podiatr Med Surg
23 (2006) xi–xiii

CLINICS IN
PODIATRIC
MEDICINE AND
SURGERY

Foreword

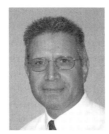

Vincent J. Mandracchia, DPM, MS
Consulting Editor

After a time, you may find that "having"

is not so pleasing a thing, after all, as "wanting."

It is not logical, but it is often true.

—Mr. Spock (*Star Trek*, "Amok Time," 1967)

I am constantly amazed at the volume of articles that medical students copy—they can amass an incredible article library in just 4 years. However, I am often interested in how little they actually read. This seems to be the way with many things. We see, and we compare, rightly or wrongly, and we want whatever we see. We don't always think about the ramifications of what it is that we desire. More importantly, we don't necessarily prepare for what it is that we desire.

I believe that our profession provides wonderful opportunities for a fulfilling and rewarding career. Yet we are still in a 1970s frame of mind regarding podiatry. We have made no significant strides in communicating to incoming students that podiatry is a versatile field—that you can be a generalist or a pediatric, diabetic, or sports medicine specialist and be successful. For example, I marvel at the strides our profession has made in the area of diabetic foot care. Certainly, we are recognized as the premier lower extremity specialists when treating patients with diabetes—but it goes much further than that. We as physicians (a status that we "wanted" and fought for) are

doi:10.1016/j.cpm.2006.05.006

expected to be knowledgeable in the recognition and immediate treatment of a patient's fluctuating blood sugar. This is an example of the "having." We have attained an important status, but we rarely make this known to potential podiatry students.

There is no doubt that surgery, with all its rights and privileges, is exciting and in many cases desirable; however, not every podiatric medical student is necessarily "surgeon material." Yet this is the area of podiatry that is exalted by the profession. I have no problem with that, but I believe that podiatry is so much more. We need to attract students that are interested in this "so much more." For example, we need research-oriented students. We need students that desire to be podiatric generalists or geriatric specialists. We need students who can be pediatric specialists.

Many in our profession feel that because podiatry is by its very nature a specialty that further specialization is neither possible nor lucrative. I disagree. At the University of Iowa, we give our residents the opportunity to rotate and interact with Ignacio Ponseti, MD. Dr. Ponseti limits his practice to the treatment of clubfoot deformity and is extremely busy. He has patients visit him from around the world because of his expertise and reputation. Why do we feel that this type of situation is not available to podiatrists? Interestingly, Dr. Ponseti is considering retirement (remarkably at age 92 he is still quite active), and has expressed regret that no one in the Orthopedics Department at the University of Iowa is interested in continuing his work. Here is an opportunity for podiatry to continue this work, yet this opportunity is not limited to Iowa alone.

To foster these opportunities, we need to attract desirable students to pursue these interests. This will be possible only if we expand the profession and let it be known that these opportunities exist. If we tout only surgery, then we will miss the chance to attract these "other" students and miss an opportunity to expand the field of podiatry to what it can and should be. Furthermore, logic dictates that expanding the profession will have the obvious benefit of more intraprofessional referrals and, subsequently, better patient care.

There is no worse feeling than facing a resident in a 3-year surgical training program who does not belong there and probably does not want to be there, who is struggling, and who we know will never be a surgeon. This student came to podiatry school thinking, even hoping, that they would be a surgeon from the get-go, because that is how the profession is viewed. This same student may indeed have the potential to be a great podopediatrician or podiatric medical generalist, but may consider the pursuit of that avenue to be less desirable and themselves a failure.

Lets stop turning potential qualified students away who either don't want to be or feel that they can't be surgeons, and lets promote podiatry for what it is in its entire depth and breadth. Knowing that our profession provides wonderful opportunities to affect patients in so many positive ways, with so many different specialties, is the true "having" that rewards one for life.

Vincent J. Mandracchia, DPM, MS
Broadlawns Medical Center
1801 Hickman Road
Des Moines, IA 50314, USA

E-mail address: vmandracchia@broadlawns.org

Clin Podiatr Med Surg
23 (2006) xv–xvii

CLINICS IN
PODIATRIC
MEDICINE AND
SURGERY

ELSEVIER
SAUNDERS

Preface

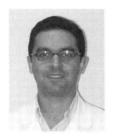

Babak Baravarian, DPM
Guest Editor

It is truly a pleasure to act as a guest editor for an issue that I believe carries far more controversy than it should. The concept of peripheral nerve surgery has always had a stigma associated with it that makes the surgical procedures seem unnecessary and unlikely to truly help the patient. My interest in peripheral nerve surgery was brought about by my poor outcomes as a resident and as an early practitioner. I did not know how to properly care for many of the patients who I would see with generalized lower extremity pain, diabetic nerve pain, neuroma pain, and tarsal tunnel. I sometimes found that neuroma nerve resections did not work well and even caused an increase in general foot pain. Tarsal tunnel syndrome was very difficult for me to treat and often frustrated me greatly with or without surgery. Diabetic neuropathy was a dilemma that had no answer and many of my patients begged me for treatments I did not know how to provide. Finally, idiopathic peripheral neuropathy, generalized nerve pain, and lower extremity nerve pain, such as reflex sympathetic dystrophy, brought an immediate referral to the pain clinic when I first started in practice. I often thought that the patients were difficult, had seen many physicians with no resolution, and had symptoms that did not make sense so they could not be real. My frustrations lead me to research and I met Dr. Dellon at a lecture that I was giving. I heard him give a talk on peripheral nerve surgery in diabetic patients and his overall results, and was hooked. With time and 2 years of additional research, I began to understand that his ideas made sense. Why cut out a neuroma in the foot when it is not done as a primary treatment in any other region of the body? Is the nerve really scarred and

0891-8422/06/$ - see front matter © 2006 Elsevier Inc. All rights reserved.
doi:10.1016/j.cpm.2006.05.001
podiatric.theclinics.com

damaged or just compressed and swollen? I began simply by decompressing neuromas instead of cutting them out. What a difference. One week of recovery, no pain, and no stump neuromas. Furthermore, in the rare case a patient still had some pain, I still could cut the nerve out or use alcohol to sclerose the nerve, leaving my options open. However, most patients had such relief of pain, they did not want any further treatment. I then decided to take Dr. Dellon's course. After a few days with him in Baltimore, I felt like a whole world had been opened to me. I began to think back to all the patients I could have helped if I had known this material sooner and decided that I would share the information with my colleagues as soon as I felt comfortable with the information. Two years have now gone by since my last visit to Baltimore and I feel that peripheral nerve surgery is the least understood, the least taught, and the least accepted area of foot and ankle surgery. However, all pain relates to nerve pain. Therefore a conceptual understanding of nerve pain and peripheral nerve surgery can help in regular care of all foot and ankle conditions, not to mention those patients with symptoms that do not make sense to you at the present time.

Today, I believe 20% of my practice focuses on peripheral nerve problems. Most of the patients have diabetic nerve pain, local compression syndromes, or misdiagnoses of reflex sympathetic dystrophy because of a lack of understanding of what the actual problem with their foot condition is. I get referrals from the pain clinic instead of referring to the pain clinic, and I am looking forward to seeing peripheral nerve problems instead of turning them away. A word of caution to all those interested in peripheral nerve surgery: take it slow and learn all the subtle details of the surgeries in order to perform the perfect procedure. With peripheral nerve surgery, you cannot have a fairly good surgery, you have to have a perfect surgery. Unlike bone surgery, the nerves are not happy unless they are fully happy. Take care and you will be well rewarded with happy patients. I highly suggest Dr. Dellon's peripheral nerve surgery workshop as an initial guide and early teaching platform, and I wish all of you luck.

This issue begins with an article by the father of modern peripheral nerve surgery, A. Lee Dellon, MD. Dr. Dellon has published so many articles on peripheral nerve surgery including more basic science research than I could ever imagine a clinical physician being able to perform. Although the article is historical in nature, it shows how truly happy he is that his life struggle with the acceptance of his techniques has begun to materialize and physicians are beginning to embrace his art and scientific expertise. There are two articles on nerve testing: one on Electromyelogram (EMG) and nerve conduction (NCV) testing and the other on pressure specified neurosensory testing (PSSD). Both of these tests have a place in my practice and truly help with patient care. I prefer the use of the PSSD test as it is not painful and can be repeated easily. I have found the information for sensory nerve testing equally good from each test, the NCV and PSSD, and excellent when combined. The testing articles are followed by a list of topics related to nerve surgery and one final article on physical therapy of peripheral nerve surgery. In whole, I hope the articles help act as a teaching guide to students, residents, physicians, and patients. I would like to thank my wife and children, Haley and Michael, for their patience, and Dr. Dellon and his staff for their assistance and tutelage. I believe peripheral nerve surgery is an infant about to grow up and I am truly excited to help it mature. With increased testing modalities including imaging of peripheral nerves and ever-improving surgical procedures, the future is bright for the treatment and outcomes of peripheral nerve pain.

Babak Baravarian, DPM
The Foot and Ankle Institute of Santa Monica
2121 Wilshire Boulevard, Suite 101
Santa Monica, CA 90403, USA

E-mail address: bbaravarian@mednet.ucla.edu

ELSEVIER
SAUNDERS

Clin Podiatr Med Surg
23 (2006) 497–508

CLINICS IN
PODIATRIC
MEDICINE AND
SURGERY

From There to Here: A Personal Viewpoint after Three Decades of Neuropathy Research

A. Lee Dellon, MD

Suite 370, 3333 North Calvert St., Baltimore, Maryland, 21218, USA

Currently there is unprecedented interested in research, writing, and clinical experience related to lower extremity peripheral nerve surgery. Its time is here, now. Box 1 lists many events from 2005 alone that support this notion. It has been my privilege and honor to have a leadership role in this awareness.

How did I get here from there?

When I graduated from medical school at Johns Hopkins University in 1970, there was a war in Vietnam. I was among the luckiest of young doctors. Five were chosen from the United States of America to be clinical associates in the National Institutes of Health, National Cancer Institute, Surgery Branch. My clinical associate position was to begin after I had completed 2 years of general surgery training at Columbia-Presbyterian Hospital in New York City. I was to be a lieutenant commander in the United States Health Service.

In medical school, I knew I was destined to be a plastic surgeon and loved research. My early clinical studies involved the mechanism of cleft palate speech and evaluation of sensibility in the hand. By the end of medical school, I had (1) suggested a new operation to correct the anatomic abnormality of the levator veli palatini muscle that was the basis for most velopharyngeal incompetence and cleft palate hearing loss, (2) defined the sequence of sensory recovery for the large myelinated touch fibers, and (3) described the method of sensory re-education for the problems related to

The author has a proprietary interest in the Pressure-Specified Sensory Device.
E-mail address: ALDellon@DellonInstitute.com

Box 1. It is the best of times

For those of us interested in the peripheral nerve, consider the
positive indicators for this field just in 2005.
The December 2005 issue of *Clinics in Podiatric Medicine and
Surgery*, for the first time is devoted to peripheral nerve
surgery. A 1999 *Clinics in Podiatric Medicine and Surgery*
was devoted to clinical neurology (medicine) [1].
January 2005, at the 14th Annual Meeting of **the American
Society for Peripheral Nerve Surgery, Jerome Steck, DPM**,
became the second podiatric physician to present a paper to
this society. Dr Steck presented the results of his surgery to
relieve pain and restore sensation in patients with neuropathy.
Stephen L Barrett, DPM becomes associate professor at the
new **Midwestern College of Health Sciences in Phoenix**,
and begins to teach the surgery course to the new students
of podiatry. His teaching will include Dellon's book,
Somatosensory Testing and Rehabilitation [2], as one of the
textbooks for the course. His students will learn endoscopic
interdigital nerve decompression and that the symptoms of
diabetic neuropathy can be relieved by decompression of
peripheral nerves, thereby restoring balance, preventing
falls, and preventing ulceration and amputation.
The *Journal of the American Podiatric Medical Association*
had a **Special Issue on the Peripheral Nerve** [3], which
included 14 papers from the 2nd Annual Meeting of the
Peripheral Nerve Fellowship Group. Seventy-three
physicians attended that meeting, including podiatric foot
and ankle surgeons, plastic surgeons, orthopedic surgeons,
neurosurgeons, and a vascular surgeon.
At the **3rd annual meeting of the Peripheral Nerve Fellowship
Group,** participating physicians from podiatry were joined
again by those from other surgical subspecialties.
At the 20th Advanced Lower Extremity Peripheral Nerve
Workshop, three podiatric foot and ankle surgeons who work
on the **Native American, Gila Reservation, of Sacaton,
Arizona**, were trained in neurosensory testing and surgery.
The 22nd and 23rd **Advanced Lower Extremity Peripheral Nerve
Workshops** were held in Baltimore. At present more than
250 surgeons have been trained doing lower extremity
peripheral nerve surgery for painful neuromas, nerve
compression, and neuropathy in 41 states within the United
States and in 15 other countries.

At the **American College of Surgeons** annual meeting,
Dr Dellon gave a half-hour presentation, "Can we cure
diabetic neuropathy?" The subject was determined by the
program committee.

In May 2005, the Board of Trustees of the **American Podiatric
Medical Association** was petitioned to begin a Related
Organization (subsection) devoted to the peripheral nerve.
The name of the subsection as proposed is The **American
Association of Lower Extremity Peripheral Nerve Surgeons**.
There were 123 names were on the application.

At the annual meeting of **American College of Foot and Ankle
Surgery**, two separate sessions were devoted to the
peripheral nerve. In one of these, **Christopher T. Maloney,
Jr., MD**, presented the results of his first 200 nerve
decompressions in patients with neuropathy. At the same
meeting a similar talk by **Kent DiNucci, DPM**, was picked up
by the local CBS affiliate, giving this story widespread
representation in the media. Dr DiNucci presented his first
72 patients with this approach to neuropathy.

Numerous books and book chapters were published in 2005
with chapters related to Dr Dellon's approach to peripheral
nerve surgery [4–16].

The **American Association of Indian Physicians** sponsored
a full workshop entitled **"Diabetic Neuropathy: Together
We Can Change its Natural History."** The workshop was
attended by American Indians from tribes across the United
States and physicians from the Indian Health Service.

Marcus Castro Fereirra, MD, Chief of Plastic Surgery at the
University of Sao Paolo, Brazil, presented his own results
using Dr Dellon's approach to decompression of lower
extremity peripheral nerves. This was presented to the
National Plastic Surgery Society of Mexico in Vera Cruz.

In **Istanbul, Turkey**, a three day Lower Extremity Peripheral
Nerve Workshop was held. This was organized by **Fuat
Yuksel**, MD, a Professor of Plastic Surgery in Istanbul, who
independently corroborated Dr Dellon's basic science work
on diabetic rats, and demonstrated the value of adding the
internal neurolysis.

**The Dellon Institute for Peripheral Nerve Surgery opened in
Boston. Virginia Hung, MD**, is the Director of the Boston
Dellon Institute. She did a Hand Surgery Fellowship at Union
Memorial Hospital in Baltimore and then additional
peripheral nerve surgery training with Dr. Dellon.

Gedge D. Rosson, MD became the second person to complete a 1 year **Peripheral Nerve Fellowship** with Dr. Dellon. Dr. Rosson returned to Johns Hopkins Hospital to be full-time on their faculty and do peripheral nerve surgery and research.

Ivan Ducic, MD, PhD, the first person to complete the 1 year peripheral nerve fellowship with Dr. Dellon, is **Program Chair for the American Society for Peripheral Nerve Surgery**. He has published ten papers in peer-reviewed journals from the research done during that fellowship. Dr. Ducic is an assistant professor at Georgetown University in Washington, DC.

NeuropathyRegistry.com went on line. Its purpose is to make available to the public the outcomes information related to the work being done by the doctors trained at the Advanced Lower Extremity Peripheral Nerve Workshops. This database permits surgeons to enter coded, HIPPA compliant, data on outcomes of nerve decompressions on patients with neuropathy, relating to pain, sensation, ulcer, amputation, balance, pain medication. It updates in real time.

Regulatory and reimbursement issues continue to consume time from the lives of all physicians. With regard to the Pressure-Specified Sensory Device, individual podiatric physicians have been engaged by Medicare in different regions of the United States. Issues related to medical necessity and research have been raised. R*ulings in favor of the PSSD* have been obtained, two at the Medicare Level, and three at the Judiciary Law Judge level, in several different states. Neurosensory testing is the functional equivalent of electrodiagnostic testing and is critical for the physician to make treatment decisions for patient care.

Lower Extremity Peripheral Nerve Surgery, a new textbook, by A. Lee Dellon, MD was begun. It is hoped that this new book will provide the foundation for those surgeons who would like to help patients with peripheral nerve problems from the groin to the toes.

inadequate sensory nerve regeneration. I had published nine papers related to cleft palate speech and two related to nerves in the hand.

My mission in the U.S. Public Health Service was to evaluate tumor immunology in lung cancer and esophageal cancer. Because I knew that I would be a plastic surgeon, my extra-curricular research involved skin cancer and peripheral nerve regeneration. My first microsurgical repairs (of subhuman primate median nerves) were done in the Surgery Branch of the National Cancer Institute. By dividing the nerves first, I was able to show degeneration of Meissner Corpuscles in the fingertip pulp, and then, by repairing the nerves, I was able to demonstrate that the old corpuscles became re-innervated, and that they did not generate de novo. I won national research prizes related to (1) predicting survival from lung cancer related to changes in the host T-cell levels during radiation therapy, (2) predicting recurrence of positive margin basal and squamous cell carcinoma related to the host cellular response to the tumor, and (3) proving that a sensory corpuscle could be re-innervated in a subhuman primate model. From my 2 years in Bethesda, Maryland, 23 papers would ultimately be published in the fields of general surgery, obstetrics and gynecology, urology, ophthalmology, dermatology, surgical oncology, and plastic surgery.

In 1974, I returned to The Johns Hopkins Hospital, where I spent 4 more years training. I completed general surgery training sufficiently to undertake my plastic surgery residency, in the middle of which, I spent time completing my hand fellowship. I spent 8 years in training after medical school. I had prepared to be a department chairman in plastic surgery, but such a job was not available in July 1978, so I resolved to set a course to be an academic in private practice. One day per week was set aside. Through the end of June 2005, 20% of my 27 years as a plastic surgeon has been devoted to research and teaching. In reality, because of many months spent teaching outside of Baltimore, about 30% of my time has been spent in research and teaching.

Sometime during my medical school education my mother was diagnosed with type 2 diabetes mellitus. At some subliminal level, this had to have influenced my direction and research. I remember my father telling me how he would help the burning pain in her legs by holding them tightly. In 1987, she fell and fractured her left humerus. This was corrected with a plate and screws. Afterwards my mother would rub her thumb against her left index finger to help the burning pain. She had a Tinel sign over the radial sensory nerve. I asked her doctor to do a neurolysis of this nerve; however, he suggested that because I had described that entrapment just the previous year in the *Journal of Hand Surgery* [17], I should perform my mother's surgery. And so I did. And her pain went away. In May of 1989, she sent to me pages torn from *Diabetes Forcast*, which included an article written by Dr. Peter James Dyck, a young neurologist at the Mayo Clinic. His article was entitled "Aldose Reductase Inhibitors and Diabetic Neuropathy [18]." In October, she slipped and fell at our home because she had not been able to feel the steps. She fractured her hip, which was then pinned, but suffered a pulmonary embolus the next day and died. I had not thought (perhaps not had the courage) to apply the surgery that I had been developing for lower extremity nerve decompressions to my mother. I know she would have been happy to try it for the first time. My first paper on this subject, "Optimism for Diabetic Neuropathy," was published in 1988 [19]. The results of my first clinical study on decompression of lower extremity peripheral nerves, was published in 1992 [20].

In 1994, I was promoted to full professor of surgery in the Division of Plastic Surgery, Johns Hopkins University, and received a joint appointment in the Department of Neurosurgery. I was the first person in 102 years that was promoted to full professor in surgery at that university, while in private practice.

In 1998, in response to requests from podiatric physicians on the Sells Reservation of the Tohono O'Odham Tribe of American Indians, I went to the Arizona to offer help. About 50% of this tribe has diabetes. In Arizona, 25% of the population is Hispanic and this ethnic group has an incidence of 15% diabetes. My help was needed and I stayed. I Opened an office and obtained a faculty appointment at the University of Arizona in Tucson. By July 2002, I was sufficiently busy that help was needed, and Christopher T. Maloney Jr., MD, originally from Tucson and a Harvard-trained plastic surgeon, was invited to join me. The following year, Stephen L. Barrett, DPM began to work with us in Tucson as well. Dr. Barrett was a valued faculty member of our Advanced Lower Extremity Peripheral Nerve Workshop. In Phoenix, he became associate professor of the new Midwestern School for Podiatry in late 2004.

In 2000, and concurrent with moving my office to Union Memorial Hospital, I changed the name of my practice to the Institute for Peripheral Nerve Surgery. This name change reflected the mixture of research, publishing, and patient care that was more appropriate to an Institute than a single surgeon in private practice. In 2003, Ramon DeJesus, MD, a Johns Hopkins-trained plastic surgeon, joined me in practice, about six months after the peripheral nerve fellowship was begun.

And that brings us back to here. Along the way, four books were written, more than 365 papers published in peer-reviewed journals, and more than 65 chapters were published in other people's books.

The Contrarians

Much of what I developed relating to the treatment of painful lower extremity nerve injuries and nerve compressions is now accepted: these approaches are a direct extension of what I developed for the nerve problems in the upper extremity. However, the application of nerve decompression symptoms of neuropathy remains controversial, thought provoking, and a point of contention for many people in podiatry, neurology, and general medicine. My work was inspired by diabetic patients for whom I had done either carpal or cubital tunnel decompressions. They would often comment that their hands felt so much better and ask if the same help wasn't available for their feet. It wasn't until the early 1980s that I was able to say, "Why not, maybe there are sites of nerve compression in the leg, like there are in the hand." And the rest is the history you are now reading.

In the last few years, there has been an explosion of review articles on neuropathy, its causes and treatment [21–29]. Curiously, most of these articles do not mention the advances described above. For example, in a 2004 monumental review in *Diabetes Care* Boulton and colleagues [21] cite 310 references, but not one related to peripheral nerve decompression. In a 2005 review by Singh and coworkers published in the *Journal of the American Medical Association* [27], 128 references are cited, but none of the articles in Table 1 are listed at all. Of the 25 referenced articles that relate to surgery, the operations are all related to correction of biomechanical foot problems, and none relate to decompression of peripheral nerves. It is fair to conclude from these reviews that there currently is no medically available treatment for idiopathic neuropathy or diabetic neuropathy. The various

Table 1
Diabetic neuropathy: results of posterior tibial nerve decompression

Study	Number of		Improvement	
	Patients	Nerves	Pain	Sensibility
1992, Dellon [7]	22	31	85%	72%
1995, Wieman & Patel[a]	33	26	92%	72%
2000, Caffee[b]	58	36	86%	50%
2000, Aszmann et al.[c]	16	12	NA	69%
2001, Tambwekr[d]	10	10	80%	70%
2003, Wood & Wood[e]	33	33	90%	70%
2004, Biddinger & Amend[f]	15	22	86%	80%
2004, Valdivia et al.[g]	60	60	85%	85%
2004, Lee & Dellon[h]	46	46	92%	92%
2005, Steck[i]	25	25	84%	72%
2005, Rader[j]	49	49	90%	75%
Totals	367	325	88%	78%

Abbreviation: NA, data is not available.

[a] Wieman TJ, Patel VG. Treatment of hyperesthetic neuropathic pain in diabetics; decompression of the tarsal tunnel. Ann Surg 1995;221:660–5.

[b] Chafee H. Decompression of peripheral nerves for diabetic neuropathy. Plast Reconstr Surg 2000;106:813–5.

[c] Aszmann OA, Kress KM, Dellon AL. Results of decompression of peripheral nerves in diabetics: a prospective, blinded study. Plast Reconstr Surg 2000;106:816–21.

[d] Tambwekar SR. Extended neurolysis of the posterior tibial nerve to improve sensation in diabetic neuropathic feet. Plast Reconstr Surg 2001;108:1452–3.

[e] Wood WA, Wood MA. Decompression of peripheral nerve for diabetic neuropathy in the lower extremity. J Foot Ankle Surg 2003;42:268–75.

[f] Biddinger K, Amend KA. The role of surgical decompression for diabetic neuropathy. Foot & Ankle Clin N Amer 2004;9:239–54.

[g] Valdivia JMV, Weinand M, Maloney CT Jr. Surgical treatment of peripheral neuropathy: outcomes from 100 consecutive surgical cases. Presented at the Annual Meeting of the Neurosurgical Society of the Southwest. Phoenix, Arizona, 2004.

[h] Lee C, Dellon AL. Prognostic ability of Tinel sign in determining outcome for decompression surgery in diabetic and non-diabetic neuropathy. Ann Plast Surg 2004;53:523–27.

[i] Steck JK. Results of decompression of lower extremity nerves in patients with symptomatic neuropathy of unknown etiology. Presented at the Annual Meeting of the American Society for Peripheral Nerve Surgery. Puerto Rico, January 16, 2005.

[j] Rader, A. Results of tibial nerve decompression in diabetics in terms of pain relief and recovery of sensibility. J Am Pod Med Assoc 2005;95(Sept/Oct).

hopes of aldose reductase inhibitors, myoinositol additives, insulin-like growth factors, nerve-type growth factors, growth hormone-type growth factors, and alpha-linoleic acid, have simply not been demonstrated to help patients with neuropathy. Pain management is available with neuropathic pain medications such as gabapentin or tramadol [30–32], and perhaps the new neuropathic pain medications released in 2005 by the Food and Drug Administration. Narcotics in various forms can be added to these medications. Nothing has been shown to prevent the progressive and irreversible natural course of neuropathy.

By the end of 2005, there were more than a dozen studies demonstrating that the basic neuropathy causes metabolic changes that render the peripheral nerve susceptible to chronic nerve compressions. In the animal models, where medical treatments can reverse the electrophysiologic changes of neuropathy shortly after it begins, we have a very different situation then we have in our patients, where symptoms may be present for years before the patient is admitted into a drug study. I interpret this discrepancy between the Phase I and II (animal and efficacy/complication) versus the Phase III (clinical studies) to mean that the patients have fixed pathophysiologic changes caused by chronic nerve compression at known sites of entrapment that are beyond the ability of a metabolic change to correct. My hypothesis continues to assert that surgical decompression of known sites of compression can relieve symptoms of neuropathy that are caused by superimposed nerve compressions. Table 1 includes many independent observations on prospective cohort single surgeon series of patients. They all demonstrate the same thing: about 80% of patients experience relief of pain, 70% experience recovery of sensation, and these combine to prevent ulcer formation and amputation. Recovery of balance prevents falls and fractures.

There seems to be, however, growing among the contrarians the realization that nerve decompression does work in patients who have diabetic neuropathy. Consider this quote from a review article in late 2004 [24]:

Common entrapments involve the median, ulnar, and peroneal nerves, the lateral cutaneous of the thigh, and the tibial nerve in the tarsal canal. The entrapment neuropathies are highly prevalent in the diabetic population, one in every three patients has one, and it should be actively sought in every patient with the signs and symptoms of neuropathy because the treatment may be surgical.....In conclusion, up to one-third of patients with diabetes are found to have some form of entrapment syndrome. The diagnosis rests on an index of suspicion and electrophysiological tests demonstrating for the most part a block in nerve conduction across the site of the lesion. The value of the Tinel sign in predicting outcome needs validation, and quantitative sensory tests are notoriously unreliable. There are clear indications for surgery when conservative medical therapy fails, and it is not yet clear that decompression should be considered in the treatment of diabetic neuropathy in the absence of compression. Prospective studies on the role for decompression using accepted measures are clearly needed.

There are those who demand patient care today be guided by class I evidence, the type provided in a prospective randomized controlled study. What is it, I wonder, that surgical decompression should be randomized against? The surgeons in the Table 1 studies surely all agree that they are biased, and that surgery can be a placebo. So it is reasonable to compare the outcome of nerve decompression to a group of patients receiving the best medical and foot care. Is it reasonable, even ethical, to randomize a group of patients to having a sham operation? Certainly the results of a randomized treatment type of study, if it were to show outcomes improved with nerve decompression, would be sufficient to convert the contrarians. And what should be the outcomes? Electrical testing, certain to be requested, has serious drawbacks in that many compressed nerves never recover normal myelination when decompressed. A crucial recent study evaluated whether traditional electrodiagnostic testing could identify a superimposed nerve compression in a patient who has diabetic neuropathy, using that compression most easily diagnosed, carpal tunnel syndrome (CTS) [33]:

> The prevalence of clinical CTS was 2% in the reference population, 14% in diabetic subjects without DPN [diabetic polyneuropathy], and 30% in those with DPN. Multiple linear regression analysis revealed that mean electrodiagnostic parameters are not significant predictors of clinical CTS in patients with diabetes. Generally, the parameters worsened with severity of neuropathy, but none reliably distinguished diabetic patients with and without CTS....Given the high prevalence of CTS in patients with DPN and that electrodiagnostic criteria cannot distinguish those with clinical CTS, it is recommended that therapeutic decisions for CTS be made independently of electrodiagnostic findings...The frequency of electrophysiological and clinical CTS in diabetic subjects with and without DPN demands an etiological explanation. It is hypothesized that the median nerve is made more susceptible to the pressure effects existing in the carpal tunnel when underlying DPN, a length-dependent axonopathy, is present. The anatomy of the carpal tunnel may produce local vascular compromise, which is superimposed on the metabolically disordered nerve or a nerve with established endoneurial ischemia, leading to frequent dysfunction in this short nerve segment. This combination of insults may result in impaired axonal transport producing local pathology and retrograde nerve dysfunction.

When these new class I studies are done, outcome measures other than, or in addition to, traditional electrophysiology must be included. New quality-of-life outcome studies would be critical to include, as well as studies about decreases in pain medication, improvement in balance, a decrease in falls. To which should be added measures of large-fiber function, such as the cutaneous pressure threshold, as measured with the Pressure-Specified Sensory Device, as this is the most sensitive measurement of this function. A visual analog scale for pain should be included.

Finally, it has been said by one of the contrarians, that "The ability to manage successfully the many different manifestations of diabetic neuropathy depends ultimately on success in uncovering the pathogenic processes underlying this disorder [23]." The basic mechanisms that I described above, which render the nerve in diabetic neuropathy susceptible to compression, have been tested in an animal model of diabetes [34,35]. In perhaps the most important of my studies on the basic mechanisms involved in my hypothesis, a group of diabetic rats was created that had no site of anatomic narrowing on the tibial nerve. The ligament in the medial ankle region of the rats was microsurgically divided. These animals were followed for 1 year; their blood sugar measured ≥ 400 mg/dL. They were compared with a group of animals identical except that they had an intact tarsal tunnel. The animals without a potential site of entrapment walked like normal animals for 1 year (ie, did not develop a neuropathic walking track pattern). That research was published in 1991 and 1994. It has since been confirmed by an independent group of plastic surgeons from Turkey, led by Fuat Yuksel, MD, who demonstrated, in 2003, the value of doing an internal neurolysis [36]. That observation was again validated, by the same basic science approach, in 2005, from the laboratory of Dr. Maria Siemionow, at the Cleveland Clinic, with extension to include documentation that motor strength is also improved by the decompression procedure [37]. The basic mechanisms are known.

Finally, when a patient is referred to my practice or to surgeons I have trained, the patients come for this surgical procedure, and cannot be randomized. Decision analysis, including all of the above, permits me enthusiastically to offer this surgical approach to patients and to teach it to other surgeons. A thoughtful paper came out recently year entitled "Alternatives to Randomized Clinical Research [38]." This paper discusses why "despite its methodologic strength, the randomized trial is used relatively infrequently to address clinical questions in surgery." However, I am positive that soon there will be several class I studies in progress throughout the United States that attempt to answer this critical remaining area of doubt raised by the contrarians. This is proper and necessary to do, for certainly I am among the most enthusiastic of the biased.

References

[1] Willis JD, Spadone SJ. Clinical neurology, Clinics in Podiatric Medicine and Surgery, 1999.
[2] Dellon AL. Somatosensory testing and rehabilitation. Baltimore (MD): Institute for Peripheral Nerve Surgery; 2000.
[3] Dellon AL, editor. Peripheral nerve [special issue]. J Am Pod Med Assoc 2005;95 (Sept/Oct).
[4] Dellon AL. History of peripheral nerve surgery. In: Winn HR, editor. Youmans neurological surgery. 5th edition. Philadelphia: WB Saunders Co., 2003. p. 3798–808.
[5] Dellon AL. Nerve compression syndromes. In: Mathes S, Hentz VR, editors. Plastic surgery, vol. VII. Philadelphia: WB Saunders Co., 2005. p. 1–54.

[6] Dellon AL. Painful neuromas. In: Mathes S, Hentz VR, editors. Plastic surgery, vol. VII. Philadelphia: WB Saunders Co., 2005. p. 55–87.

[7] Dellon AL. Measuring peripheral nerve function: neurosensory testing versus electrodiagnostic testing. In: Slutsky D, editor. Atlas of the hand clinics: nerve repair and reconstruction. Philadelphia: Elsevier; 2005. p. 1–31.

[8] Dellon AL. Carpal tunnel syndrome. In: Schmidt RF, Willis WD, editors. Encyclopedic reference of pain. Berlin: Springer Verlag; 2005.

[9] Dellon AL. Thoracic outlet syndrome. In: Schmidt RF, Willis WW, editors. Encyclopedic reference of pain. Berlin: Springer Verlag; 2005.

[10] Dellon AL. Ulceration: sensory restoration in extremities. In: Schmidt RF, Willis WW, editors. Encyclopedic reference of pain. Berlin: Springer Verlag; 2005.

[11] Dellon AL. Painful scars. In: Schmidt RF, Willis WW, editors. Encyclopedic reference of pain. Berlin: Springer Verlag; 2005.

[12] Dellon AL. Compression neuropathy. In: Trumble TT, Cornwall RC, Budroff J, editors. Hand, elbow, shoulder: core knowledge in orthopaedics. Graphic World Pub; 2005. p. 234–55.

[13] Dellon AL, Mont MA. Partial denervation for the treatment of painful neuromas complicating total knee arthroplasty. In: Insall JN, Scott WN, editors. Surgery of the knee. 4th edition. Philadelphia: Churchill Livingston/Elsevier; 2005.

[14] Maloney CT Jr, Dellon AL. Innovations in peripheral nerve surgery. In: Sieminow N, editor. New techniques/technologies in plastic surgery. London: Springer-Verlag; 2005. p. 55–70.

[15] Dellon AL. Musculoskeletal system; peripheral nerve injuries and entrapment. In: Orient JM, editor. Sapira's art and science of bedside diagnosis. 3rd edition. Baltimore, MD: Lippincott Williams and Wilkens; 2005. p. 546–53.

[16] Dellon AL. The neurologic exam. Sensory testing. In: Orient JM, editor. Sapira's art and science of bedside diagnosis. 3rd edition. Baltimore, MD: Lippincott Williams and Wilkens; 2005. p. 546–53.

[17] Dellon AL, Mackinnon SE. Radial sensory nerve entrapment in the forearm. J Hand Surg 1986;11A:199–205.

[18] Dyck JP. Aldose reductase inhibitors and diabetic neuropathy. Diabetes Forcast 1989.

[19] Dellon AL. Optimism in diabetic neuropathy. Ann Plast Surg 1988;20:103–5.

[20] Dellon AL. Treatment of symptoms of diabetic neuropathy by peripheral nerve decompression. Plast Reconstr Surg 1992;89:689–97.

[21] Boulton AJM, Arezzo JC, Malik RA, et al. Diabetic somatic neuropathies. Diabetes Care 2004;27:1458–86.

[22] Vinik AI. Advances in diabetes for the millennium: new treatments for diabetic neuropathies. Med Gen Med 2004;6:13–9.

[23] Vinik AI, Mehrabyan A. Diabetic neuropathies. Med Clin N Amer 2004;88:947–99.

[24] Vinik AI, Mehrabyan A, Colen L, et al. Focal entrapment neuropathies in diabetes. Diabetes Care 2004;27:1783–8.

[25] Tesfaye S, Chaturvedi N, Eaton SEM, et al. Vascular risk factors and diabetic neuropathy. N Eng J Med 2005;352:341–50.

[26] Koller H, Kiesseier BC, Jander S, et al. Chronic inflammatory demyelinating polyneuropathy. N Engl J Med 2005;352:1243–356.

[27] Singh N, Armstrong DG, Lipsky BA. Preventing foot ulcers in patients with diabetes. JAMA 2005;293:217–28.

[28] Witzke KA, Vinik AI. Diabetic neuropathy in older adults. Rev Endocr Metab Disord 2005; 6:117–27.

[29] Boulton AJM, Vinik AI, Arezzo JC, et al. Diabetic neuropathies: a statement by the American Diabetes Association. Diabetes Care 2005;28:956–62.

[30] Gilron I, Bailey JM, Tu D, et al. Morphine, Gabapentin, or their combination for neuropathic pain. N Engl J Med 2005;352:1324–34.

[31] Raja SN, Haythornwaite JA. Combination therapy for neuropathic pain: which drugs, which combination, which patients? N Engl J Med 2005;352:1373–5.

[32] Raskin P, Donofrio PD, Rosenthal NR, et al. Topiramate vs placebo in painful diabetic neuropathy: analgesic and metabolic effects. Neurology 2004;63:865–73.

[33] Perkins B, Olaleye D, Bril V. Carpal tunnel syndrome in patients with diabetic polyneuropathy. Diabetes Care 2002;25:565–9.

[34] Dellon ES, Dellon AL. Functional assessment of neurologic impairment: track analysis in diabetic and compression neuropathies. Plast Reconstr Surg 1991;88:686–94.

[35] Dellon ES, Dellon AL, Seiler WA IV. The effect of tarsal tunnel decompression in the streptozotocin-induced diabetic rat. Microsurg 1994;15:265–8.

[36] Kale B, Yuksel F, Celikoz B, et al. Effect of various nerve decompression procedures on the functions of distal limbs in streptozotocin-induced diabetic rats: further optimism in diabetic neuropathy. Plast Reconstr Surg 2003;111:2265–72.

[37] Demir Y, Sari A, Siemionow M. Impact of early decompression on development of superimposed neuropathy in diabetic rats. Presented at the Annual Meeting of the American Association for Surgery of the Hand. Puerto Rico, January 15, 2005.

[38] Graham B. Alternatives to randomized trials in clinical research. J Am Soc Surg Hand 2005; 5:61–8.

ELSEVIER
SAUNDERS

Clin Podiatr Med Surg
23 (2006) 509–530

CLINICS IN
PODIATRIC
MEDICINE AND
SURGERY

Conservative Treatment of Peripheral Neuropathy and Neuropathic Pain

David A. Francis, DPM[a], Anne T. Christopher, MD[b],
Bradley D. Beasley, DPM[c],*

[a]Green Country Podiatry Center, 3647 South Harvard, Tulsa, OK 74133-2227, USA
[b]Pain Evaluation & Treatment Center, 5801 East 41st Street, Suite 1000,
Tulsa, OK 74135-3888, USA
[c]Metro Tulsa Foot & Ankle Specialists, 421 West Washington,
Broken Arrow, OK 74012, USA

"On either foot the soles were burning; whence the flexile joints glanced with such violent writhes. As flame, feeding on unctuous matter, glides along the surface, scarcely touching where it moves; so here, from heel to point, glided the flames."

— Dante Alighieri in The Divine Comedy

Fortunately, most conditions treated by physicians can be easily visualized, palpated, quantified, or clearly described by the patient. Symptoms associated with peripheral neuropathy lack these characteristics and provide a constant challenge for physicians who encounter the sequelae of neuropathy. During the past decade, a growing arsenal of treatment options offers relief for both frustrated clinicians and their patients whose quality of life has been negatively impacted by this condition. Unfortunately, the flood of new treatment modalities can create a confusing menu for physicians.

There are many types of peripheral nerve disorders that lead to peripheral neuropathy, and estimates suggest that at least 1.5% of the U.S. population suffers from symptomatic neuropathy [1]. The most common identifiable etiology of neuropathy in the western world is diabetes [2]. Interestingly, neuropathy is the most common complication associated with diabetes and leads to the highest incidence of morbidity [3]. For example, neuropathy increases the risk of amputation nearly twofold. Moreover, the presence of diabetic peripheral neuropathy (DPN) and deformity leads to a 12-fold

* Corresponding author.
E-mail address: brad.beasley@cox.net (B.D. Beasley).

0891-8422/06/$ - see front matter © 2006 Elsevier Inc. All rights reserved.
doi:10.1016/j.cpm.2006.04.004   podiatric.theclinics.com

increase in amputation risk and a 36-fold increased risk if there is a history of ulceration [4]. In the United States, 85,000 amputations are performed each year, one every 10 minutes, and neuropathy is considered to be the major contributor in 87% of the cases. Amputation obviously decreases quality of life for the patient and can lead to mortality within 5 to 10 years for nearly 50% of these patients. Even if wound complications do not result from DPN, approximately 10% of these neuropathy patients experience persistent pain [5].

This review simplifies the application of non-surgical treatment options for symptomatic peripheral neuropathy. Diabetic peripheral neuropathy will be emphasized, because this condition is seen daily by physicians who treat the foot and ankle, and as mentioned, is the most common etiology. However, many of the discussed treatment options have equal application for neuropathies not associated with diabetes.

The frustrating and recalcitrant nature of neuropathic pain has precipitated many "alternative" treatments available to patients directly or by prescription from physicians who are exasperated with more traditional therapies. The authors can only recommend treatment modalities that have been clinically assessed with controlled trials. However, other non-traditional therapies, such as some topical treatments, have anecdotally shown excellent results and will also be discussed. Although many of the prescribed medications reviewed are being used off indication, a plethora of information exists to support their use. The onus lies with the prescribing physician to use treatments with which they are comfortable, for which they are able to monitor progress and complications, and for which they clearly understand the contraindications and interactions.

Differential diagnosis

The significance of the diabetic etiology of peripheral neuropathy is easy to recognize when one considers that nearly 1 in 10 American adults has diabetes. Prevalence of neuropathy in these patients ranges from 25% to 100%. The World Health Organization estimates that 220 million people will have diabetes worldwide by 2010 [6].

Many other causes of neuropathy exist and should be considered during the initial patient evaluation. Traumatic and entrapment neuropathies are common and often temporary. For example, neuropraxia can occur in peripheral nerves during everyday activities or simply from inappropriate shoe wear, but are usually unilateral. Severe trauma and spinal cord injuries can cause permanent sensory and motor neurodeficits. Congenital conditions such as Charcot-Marie-Tooth disease are characterized by a progressive destruction of peripheral nerves along with weakness and muscle atrophy.

Inflammatory and infectious neuropathies comprise a large group of neuropathies worldwide, but are rarer in the United States. Some of these conditions include sarcoidosis, leprosy, Lyme disease, and AIDS. Neoplastic causes of neuropathies can include carcinomas, paraneoplastic syndromes, multiple myeloma, leukemia, lymphomas, and amyloidosis. Interestingly, a few of the medications used to treat some of these conditions, especially the platinum based drugs, are also commonly responsible for toxic etiologies of neuropathy. Other toxic causes include heavy metals (lead, mercury, and arsenic), alcohol use, and hydrocarbon exposure.

Metabolic conditions other than diabetes can also lead to the development of neuropathy. Some of these conditions include uremia, pernicious anemia (B12 deficiency), hypothyroidism, hypercholesterolemia, and porphyria. A final class of related conditions involves autoimmune dysfunctions such as phospholipid antibody syndrome, chronic inflammatory demyelinating neuropathy, multifocal motor neuropathy, and Guillain-Barré syndrome [7].

The primary risk factor for DPN is hyperglycemia [8]. Studies have also shown that regular swings in blood glucose levels can precipitate the formation of neuropathy. Other risk factors, when coupled with diabetes, include cigarette smoking, alcohol consumption, hypertension, hypercholesterolemia, hypertriglyceridemia, compression, height, and advancing age [9].

Treatment options

Pharmacologic therapy

Pharmacologic management of pain associated with diabetic peripheral neuropathy must be rational and balanced. The underlying pathophysiology of diabetic neuropathy and the mechanism of action of each drug used must be evaluated each time pharmacologic therapy is being considered. The overall goal of therapy is to administer drugs that use different mechanisms of action and that will cause broad and balanced analgesic effects in treated individuals.

Diabetes is a systemic illness, which causes widespread morbidity in individuals who have the disease. Management of diabetic sequelae commonly requires effected individuals to take multiple drugs. Careful attention to side effects and potential drug-to-drug interactions is necessary at all times. Potential interactions should guide the clinician toward appropriate analgesic therapies. Metabolism and excretion of pain medication may be impaired because of compromised renal function and dosage adjustments may be necessary if creatinine clearance has been impaired. The complexity of diabetes must be understood by the practitioner who endeavors to use either pharmaceuticals approved by the Food and Drug Administration (FDA) or non-FDA-approved pharmaceuticals to manage diabetic patients.

Gabapentin (Neurontin)

Gabapentin is a gamma aminobutyric (GABA) analog. It has been used to treat neuropathic pain for 20 years but is actually indicated by the FDA as an anticonvulsant. Prospective randomized trials are underway for the treatment of diabetic neuropathy. It is now available in generic form.

The mechanism of action to block neuropathic pain is not known, but gabapentin is known to block calcium conduction through voltage-gated calcium channels at the nerve cell membrane. This action limits afferent neuronal stimulation and increases inhibitory feedback by GABA [10].

Gabapentin has few drug interactions and low toxicity. It has 13 significant side effects including dizziness, ataxia, and somnolence. Side effects are known to be dose related and can be self-limited. Gradual dose escalation can decrease the incidence of side effects. The therapeutic dose range for diabetic neuropathy is unknown and reported effective doses vary widely. Treatment ranges are from 300 mg three times a day to 1200 mg three times a day for diabetic neuropathy [10].

Tricyclic antidepressants

Common tricyclic antidepressants used for the treatment of diabetic neuropathy include amitriptyline (Elavil) and nortriptyline (Aventyl, Pamelor). Randomized studies have demonstrated statistically significant pain reduction with these agents, although they are not FDA indicated for the treatment of neuropathic pain.

Amitriptyline dosages for treatment of neuropathic pain can range from 25 mg to 150 mg daily. This drug is a tertiary amineand and was originally indicated for the treatment of depressive states. It is active in the central nervous system where it blocks sodium channels and may block N-methyl-D-aspartate (NMDA) receptors in the synaptic membranes of nerve cells [11]. Sodium channel blockade nonselectively inhibits reuptake of norepinephrine and serotonin which potentiates transmission of these neurochemicals. Although increased transmission in the central nervous system improves major depressive symptoms, it also may increase transmission in descending inhibitory pain pathways. Augmentation of descending inhibition blocks ascending pain signal propagation.

Amitriptyline is strongly antimuscarinic; individuals who have cardiac abnormalities should use the agent with caution because it may cause the development of cardiac conduction disturbances. Other common untoward effects from this drug include dry mouth, blurred vision, weight gain, and orthostatic hypotension. Individuals who have urinary retention, glaucoma, and liver disorders should also use the drug with caution.

Nortriptyline is an active metabolite of amitriptyline and has been shown to be equally effective in treating neuropathic pain with roughly half the dose equivalent of amitriptyline [12]. Secondary amines such as nortriptyline usually exhibit fewer anticholinergic affects and are better tolerated than tertiary amines, but do carry the same precautions and untoward effects. Effective nortriptyline dosages to treat neuropathic pain vary between 10 mg and 100 mg daily. Serum levels must be monitored when dosages exceed 100 mg per day. Both secondary and tertiary amines are contraindicated with mono-amine oxidase inhibitors (MAOI).

Duloxetine (Cymbalta)

Duloxetine was approved for use in September 2004 and is the first FDA-approved medication to treat diabetic neuropathic pain. Two prospective, randomized 12-week trials have demonstrated the efficacy of duloxetine for treating diabetic neuropathic pain [13–15]. In both studies, dosages of 60 mg daily and 60 mg twice daily showed efficacy in reducing pain; however, the 120 mg dose was not statistically better than the 60 mg dose. In both studies, significant pain relief, defined as a 30% reduction in the Lickert pain scale, was seen after 1 week. Improvements in pain scores escalated weekly and were sustained through the entire study. Secondary outcomes studied included pain interference, quality of life measures, and reported night pain. In these secondary measures, duloxetine given in 60 mg and 120 mg doses resulted in significantly greater improvement at study end. Once again, the 120 mg dose was not significantly different than the 60 mg dose [13–15].

Duloxetine selectively inhibits the reuptake of serotonin and norepineph-rine in a fairly balanced ratio [16]. Potentiation of serotonin and norepi-nephrine from increased concentrations causes enhanced inhibition of descending neuroregulatory pain pathways in the central nervous system. Pain reduction occurs much more quickly than mood enhancement in the 60 mg and 120 mg doses [13–15].

Data from both studies indicate side effects are dose related. Discontinu-ance rates because of adverse effects at the 60 mg dose were 14% versus 18% at the 120 mg dose. The most common side effects were mild to moderate nausea. Dizziness, somnolence, and fatigue were also commonly reported ef-fects. This drug is metabolized through the CYP2D6 enzyme pathway. Cau-tion must be used when administering this drug with other drugs that have similar metabolism, such as amitriptyline and tramadol.

Duloxetine is contraindicated with MAOI and in patients who have un-controlled narrow-angle glaucoma. Doses may be adjusted in patients who have impaired renal function (creatinine clearance < 30 mL/min) but should be avoided in end stage renal failure and in patients who have any hepatic insufficiency [17].

Venlafaxine (Effexor)

Venlafaxine also selectively blocks reuptake of norepinephrine and sero-tonin. At doses below 100 mg it has more actively increases serotonin levels but, in doses above 100 mg, it has increased levels of norepinephrine recep-tor uptake inhibition. It has not been FDA approved for the treatment of neuropathic pain but data from blinded randomized controlled crossover studies have shown venlafaxine to be as effective for treating painful poly-neuropathy as some tricyclic antidepressants [11].

Doses of venlafaxine for treating pain vary, but can range from 75 mg per day to 300 mg per day. Adverse effects include gastrointestinal upset, weight gain, sedation, and erectile dysfunction.

Pregabalin (Lyrica)

Pregabalin was approved for the treatment of diabetic neuropathic pain in January 2005. Structurally, pregabalin is an alpha2-delta ligand and an analog of GABA. It binds to the alpha2-delta subunit on the voltage-gated calcium channels at the nerve cell membrane. This binding blocks calcium influx, which reduces the release of neurotransmitters such as substance P, glutamate, and norepinephrine. Reducing these excitatory neurotransmitters is the mechanism by which pregabalin is thought to exert its analgesic effect. It has also been shown to have anxiolytic and anticonvulsant activity through the same mechanism. Despite its name, the drug has no activity at either GABA (A) or GABA (B) receptors. It has no gabanergic activity.

Rosenstock and colleagues [18] performed a prospective, double-blind, randomized trial comparing pregabalin to placebo in patients who had diabetic peripheral neuropathy. Medication dosing in the treatment arm of the study was set at 300 mg per day (100 mg three times a day). Mean endpoint pain scores were significantly reduced at 1 week in the pregabalin group and remained reduced throughout the study. Secondary outcome measures demonstrated decreased sleep interference, mood disturbance, and improved quality of life as measured by the SF-36 Health Survey in the treatment group. Approximately 10% of the treatment group withdrew because of adverse effects of the medication. These effects included somnolence, dizziness, and peripheral edema. Side effects begin as early as 1 day after the onset of treatment but may diminish over time [18].

Sharma and coworkers [19] also conducted a double-blind, placebo study on patients who had diabetic peripheral neuropathy. They used a dosage of pregabalin 150 mg per day or 600 mg per day versus placebo in three-times-a-day divided doses. Compared with placebo, the 600-mg-per-day dosage group had superior outcomes in pain reduction as well as secondary measures, which included sleep interference, quality of life, and mood. Patients withdrew at a higher rate in the 600-mg-per-day group (8.5%) because of adverse events, than in the 150-mg-per-day or placebo group, which had drop out rates of 2.5% and 4.7% respectively. In a similar study, Lesser and colleagues [20] looked at mean pain score reduction in patients receiving pregabalin 75 mg, 300 mg, or 600 mg per day in three-times-a-day divided doses. In the groups receiving pregabalin 300 mg per day and 600mg per day, a mean pain score reduction of 30% was seen in 62% and 65% respectively, which was significantly better than placebo. The 600-mg-per-day group had a significantly higher proportion of patients who achieved at least 70% pain reduction compared with any of the other groups. Patients treated with 75 mg per day did not have a significantly improved mean pain score compared with the placebo group. The most common adverse events were dizziness, somnolence, and peripheral edema. Drop out rates of 3.7%, 12.2%, and 3.1% was seen in the pregabalin 300-mg-per-day, 600-mg-per-day, and placebo groups respectively [20].

Other placebo-controlled randomized studies done on patients who had similar types of neuropathic pain have shown similarly positive results [21,22]. Dose ranges in these studies were 150 mg, 300 mg or 600 mg per day in divided doses. Quality of life improvements were seen in the treated patients at all doses in the Sabatowski study [22] but, this outcome was not duplicated in the Dworkin study [21]. Pain reduction and mood disturbance were positively effected in the treatment groups that received at least 300 mg a day. Decreased sleep interference was noted in all treatment groups. The most common adverse events were dizziness, somnolence, peripheral edema, headache, and dry mouth. The appearance of adverse events was dose related but at the 300 mg level most patients rated their adverse effects as mild or moderate in intensity.

Tramadol (Ultram)

Tramadol is a centrally acting synthetic opiate which appears to have at least two distinct mechanisms of action for alleviating pain. It binds to mu receptors throughout the central nervous system and blocks pain perception. It has been useful historically to treat nociceptive pain by this mechanism. Tramadol is also known to block monoamine transporter reuptake at the nerve cell junction in the dorsal horn, similar to tricyclic antidepressants. This is the mechanism by which tramadol has been hypothesized to have an effect on neuropathic pain [23].

There have been few studies that look at tramadol prospectively using a randomized and double-blind design, and the size of the studies have been relatively small. Meta-analysis of pooled data by Duhmke and colleagues [24] shows that tramadol is an effective treatment of neuropathic pain. A total of 161 participants were studied. In the Tramadol treatment group, 50% pain reduction was reached at a number needed to treat of 3.5. In one small, double-blind randomized trial, subcategories of pain such as allodynia and mechanical pain were found to have improved in the tramadol treatment group compared with placebo [25].

Lidocaine patch (Lidoderm)

A 5% lidocaine patch has been available for the treatment of post-herpetic neuralgia for many years. A recent prospective trial has shown that it is effective for the treatment of pain associated with diabetic neuropathy [26].

Lidocaine is an amide type local anesthetic which blocks ion channels on the neuronal cell membrane and prevents the conduction of sensory neuron action potentials. In the patch preparation, 5% lidocaine is mixed into an adhesive and applied to polyester felt backing. Each adhesive patch contains 700 mg of lidocaine in an aqueous base that facilitates transfer and absorption of the active chemical across the skin. Absorption of lidocaine is directly related to surface area upon which it is applied and the duration of the application. When worn according to dosing instructions, blood plasma concentrations of lidocaine reach approximately 0.13 μg/mL and lidocaine concentrations do not increase or accumulate with daily use [27].

The patch must be applied to intact skin because absorption rates are less predictable and could cause higher blood concentration levels. Lidocaine is metabolized in the liver and excreted by the kidney. Caution must be used with patients who have hepatic disease because of the possible accumulation of active lidocaine caused by impaired metabolism of the drug. History of drug allergy to amide anesthetics is an absolute contraindication to use of lidocaine patches [27].

A recent prospective, open-label study of 56 patients showed good efficacy of the 5% lidocaine patch for treating pain associated with diabetic peripheral neuropathy. Outcome measures included the Brief Pain Inventory (BPI), McGill Pain Questionnaire, Beck Depression Inventory (BDI), and Profile of Mood States (POMS). Hemoglobin A1C and lidocaine levels were followed throughout the study. The study lasted 3 weeks and accommodated a flexible dosing schedule: patients were allowed to wear up to four patches for a maximum of 18 hours daily. Results showed that 70% of participants had at least a 30% reduction in mean pain scores by the third week of the study. Significant improvements were also seen in the BDI and POMS scores. Pain interference scores measured in the BPI and sleep quality were also positively impacted in a significant number of individuals [26].

Nutritional supplements

From a physiologic standpoint, the path to neurotoxic destruction in the hyperglycemic state is broad and wide. Numerous machinations conspire to rob the diabetic patient of a functioning peripheral nervous system. Hyperglycemic lipid dysmetabolism which results in accelerated atherosclerosis of the vasonervorum, accumulation of advanced glycosylation end products, impaired axonal plasmic flow, the production of reactive oxidative species, reduced activity of nitric oxide synthetase, and the poisoning of the sodium potassium ATPase pump, as well as increased protein kinase C activity, all prove to be neurocidal in the uncontrolled diabetic.

The goal of nutritional therapy through dietary supplementation is to interrupt the omnibus of pathoneurophysiology at key enzymatic focal points. Naturally, nothing can supplant the normalization of the hyperglycemic state. Below is a list of nutritional supplements, some of which have been studied extensively, that can be used in the treatment of diabetic peripheral neuropathy. A functioning gastrointestinal system is paramount to the success of this therapy. Diabetic gastroparesis and syndromes will seriously preclude the efficacy of such an approach. The preferred method of absorption (parenteral versus gastrointestinal), and effective half-life of certain supplements have not been fully elucidated. Cross reactivities have not been fully studied, and current knowledge is incomplete. In some instances, effective minimal dosing has not been established. Although these supplements are thought to be relatively benign, toxic doses, if any, have not been determined. These supplements can be used individually or in combination. An overall evaluation of the patient may lead the clinician to select certain supplements to correct perceived deficiencies. Anemia, hyperlipidemia, peripheral vascular disease, and other comorbidities should be taken into account before suggesting nutritional supplementation.

Evening primrose oil

Evening primrose oil supplies gamma-linolenic acid, which improves vasodilator eicosanoid synthesis in the diabetic. This corrects nerve blood flow and nerve conduction velocity deficits, and inhibits platelet aggregation in the vasonervorum. The impairment of essential fatty acid metabolism in diabetics leads to microvascular abnormalities, neural hypoxia, and the generation of oxygen-free radicals. This process leads to endoneural damage and impaired axonal transport, as well as reduced ATPase activity [28]. Dietary supplementation of gamma-linolenic acid seems to support neuronal function and blood flow, and has shown to be successful in the reduction of neuropathic symptoms [29]. Recommended therapeutic dosages are 400 mg per day in divided doses.

Acetyl-L-carnitine

Acetyl-L-carnitine is a trimethylated amino acid that is synthesized in the human brain, liver, and kidneys. It facilitates the uptake of acetyl-CoA into the mitochondria during fatty acid oxidation, enhances acetylcholine production, and stimulates protein and membrane phospholipid synthesis [30]. In human studies where diabetic subjects received 2000 mg per day orally, results showed a statistically significant reduction of neuropathy pain (39%), improved nerve fiber regeneration, and increased nerve conduction velocities and amplitudes over a 12-month period [31,32]. Recommended dosages are 2–3 g per day in divided amounts.

Alpha lipoic acid

Alpha lipoic acid is a powerful antioxidant, scavenging hydroxy, superoxide, and peroxyl radicals. It can regenerate thioredoxin, vitamin C, and glutathione, as well as improve glucose transport in diabetics. There are several sources of oxidative stress including glycation reactions, a shift in reduced oxygen status, increased levels of lipid hydroperoxides and DNA adducts [33]. Studies indicate alpha lipoic acid is well suited for the prevention and treatment of diabetic neuropathy [34]. Studies on individuals who have type II diabetes with peripheral neuropathy, showed that when treated with intravenous alpha lipoic acid (The Sydney Trial) and oral therapy (Aladin II Trial), subjects demonstrated reduced burning, lancinating pains, and increased sensory nerve conduction velocities, as well as sensory nerve action potentials [35,36]. In vitro studies show improved endoneural blood flow and sodium-potassium ATPase activity. Alpha lipoic acid has been used in Germany since the 1960s for the treatment of neuropathic pain. When alpha lipoic acid is taken, thyroid T_3–T_4 conversions may need to be monitored, and there is the potential for hypoglycemia in well-controlled diabetics. The suggested therapeutic dosage of alpha lipoic acid is 600 mg three times daily.

Taurine

Taurine has demonstrated the ability to counteract oxidative stress and correct nerve growth factor deficits in diabetics [37]. The molecule functions as an osmolyte, calcium modulator, inhibitory neurotransmitter, and antioxidant. Studies on dietary supplementation of taurine in diabetic conditions yielded findings consistent with regulating neuronal calcium, thereby reducing nerve hyperexcitability and pain through the ascorbate system [38]. Decreased nerve blood flow and attenuated nerve growth factors were counteracted by taurine supplementation in subjects who had diabetes [37]. Suggested supplementation is 400 mg per day in divided doses.

Foltx and Metanx

Foltx comprises folic acid 2.5 mg, pyridoxine 25 mg, and cyanocobalamin 2 mg, and has been shown to lower homocysteine. There is a ninefold correlation between hyperhomocysteinemia and the development of peripheral neuropathy in diabetics. Increased homocysteine levels could impact nerve function by direct cytotoxic effects, or secondarily by oxidative damage to endothelial cells, which would lead to occlusive arteriosclerosis of the vasonervorum. Reduction of serum homocysteine levels reduces the development and symptoms of peripheral neuropathy. Foltx has been shown to significantly lower serum homocysteine. This not only reduces the incidence of atherosclerosis in the development of peripheral vascular disease, but also the development of peripheral neuropathy. Suggested Foltx dosage is one tablet per day [39].

Metanx has replaced Foltx with L-methylfolate 2.8 mg, Pyridoxal 5-Phosphate 25 mg, and methylcobalamin 2 mg. The new formulation is seven times more bioavailable because reduction steps are bypassed in metabolism. The result is superior reduction of homocysteine [40].

Magnesium

Low magnesium levels have been implicated in the role of neuropathic pain in a variety of disease states, including diabetic neuropathy. Magnesium has a positive effect on nitric oxide synthesis, N-methyl-D-aspartate receptors, and competitively inhibits calcium's role in the wind-up effect of pain perpetuation. Dietary magnesium supplementation has been shown to be beneficial in a number of chronic pain entities including migraine headaches and fibromyalgia [41].

Myo-inositol

The depletion of nerve myo-inositol has been implicated in the development of diabetic peripheral neuropathy. Oral aldose-reductase inhibitors have been used in an attempt to reverse myo-inositol depletion and reduce intracellular sorbitol accumulation, but with little success. In experimental models, supplementation of inositol in depleted disease states counteracted the decrease in associated sodium-potassium ATPase activity; it also increased nerve conduction velocity and prevented axonal atrophy [42].

Succinic acid

In a 2002 study, succinic acid's role in aerobic glycolysis has been implicated in improved basal and postprandial glycemic control, which resulted in reduction of paresthesias associated with diabetic neuropathy. Further investigations are necessary to elaborate its role in nutritional therapeutics for diabetic neuropathy [43].

Dehydroepiandrosterone

Dehydroepiandrosterone (DHEA) is reportedly reduced in diabetic states. DHEA has antioxidant properties which have shown to reduce superoxide production by epineural arterials and improve vascular relaxation, mediated by acetylcholine and increased sodium, potassium, and ATPase activity, as well as myoinositol content in nerves. The resulting endoneural blood flow corrects nerve conduction velocity impairments [44].

L-arginine

Dietary L-arginine helps to accelerate the healing of diabetic wounds, supplies nitric oxide, and functions in vasodilation. As nitric oxide synthetase is reduced in diabetics, a ready source of nitric oxide can facilitate increased endoneural blood flow. L-arginine can play an important role in helping diabetic neuropathy. Further studies are needed [45].

Benfotiamine

Benfotiamine is a lipid soluble form of vitamin B1, in the allithiamine group of naturally occurring thiamine-derived compounds. It has been shown in human endothelial studies and animal models to prevent the generation of advanced glycosylation end products (AGE). AGE has been implicated in the non-enzymatic glycation of proteins in diabetics. The result is function damage to neuronal endothelial cells, which results in vascular disturbances [46]. Placebo-controlled, double-blind studies in humans confirm a statistically significant reduction of pain in diabetics who suffer from peripheral neuropathy [47]. The recommended dosage is a 100 mg tablet four times daily. There were no observable side effects [46,47].

The complicated metabolic pathogenesis of diabetic neuropathy will certainly yield other key enzymatic deficiencies which may be corrected by exogenous supplementation. Ongoing research should give interested physicians the opportunity to correct or ameliorate this noxious malady through therapeutic nutritive modalities. Pharmacologic, naturopathic, and internet resources are invaluable as updates in the evolving armamentarium of the treatment of diabetic peripheral neuropathy.

Topical modalities

Once the diagnosis of neuropathy has been established, its etiology should be ascertained by all means possible. Successful amelioration of this condition is dependent upon therapies directed to correct the underlying cause. If the origin of the malady eludes diagnosis, symptomatic treatment can be initiated. In either case, topical therapy can be a safe primary or adjunctive therapy; untoward systemic side effects are unlikely.

Since the time of Dante's inadvertently apt description of neuropathy's tortuous pains, expeditious topical nostrums of sundry origins have been attempted. The simple act of rubbing a nociceptive nerve uses the Gate theory for pain modulation. Stimulated larger myelinated alpha nerve fiber signals in response to pressure reach the spinal cord more rapidly than the smaller unmyelinated afferent C-nociceptor fibers. The effect is interference of pain signals to the dorsal route ganglia. With the exception of certain hyperexcitable, self-reinforcing pain states, topicals are best used as adjunctive therapy to avoid drug interactions and deleterious end-organ effects. These medications also avoid first-pass metabolism by the liver. The medication is not eliminated before it reaches the target tissues. Diseases of the liver will not affect theraputic efficacies [48].

Typically topical therapies have been more successful for the treatment of superficial burning, pins and needles, coldness, and stinging dysesthesias. Centrally acting oral parenteral and intrathecal agents are used for deeper lancinating, shooting, aching pains in general.

Topical medications can be obtained as over-the-counter preparations, proprietary prescription medications, and compounded formulas. A good relationship with a local compounding pharmacist can greatly enhance a physician's therapeutic range. This modality has recently gained a considerably higher profile, because of its efficacy and safety. Below is a list of over the counter prescription and compounded topical formulas. One of the compounds, which was designed by one of the authors (D.F.) has been used since 1999 to treat painful neuralgia with relatively good success. Anecdotal reports indicate an approximately 80% success rate in the reduction of mild to moderate neurogenic pain. A wide variety of pharmaceuticals have been combined with transdermal delivery systems with variable success. The advent of new medications to treat neuropathic pain opens the door to countless combinations. The following list is meant to be instructive but not necessarily comprehensive. Although the risks of side effects and drug interactions may be minimal or negligible in many cases, relative caution should be exercised for those qualities inherent in each medication.

Over-the-counter topicals

Capsaicin

In 0.25%–0.75% preparations, this is one of the few over the counter products FDA approved for neuralgia. Capsaicin is an external analgesic derived from the Solanaceae plant family. Its mode of action involves depleting and preventing reaccumulation of substance "P" in sensory nerves. Substance "P" is a chemical pain mediator found in unmyelinated type-C neurons in the dermis and epidermis. The reduction of substance "P" in sensory neurons and inflammatory periarticular tissue reduces the perception of pain [49].

The drawback of Capsaicin is twofold. The medication itself can cause an unpleasant burning sensation with the release of substance "P" upon its application. Greater care must be exercised to avoid contact with mucous membranes, and the onset of action may take 2–6 weeks. The duration of action when the medication becomes therapeutic is 4–6 hours, which mandates frequent applications. The burning side effects may be attenuated by a combination with local topical lidocaine. This medication has been most helpful in treating neuralgic postoperative cicatrix pain. It has been effective for arthritis sufferers as well.

Biofreeze gel

Biofreeze gel is a topical 0.25% menthol gel in Ilex preparation which seems to be intermittently helpful for superficial burning dysthesias. Menthol, by inhibiting calcium currents of neuronal membranes, produces a pleasing sensation of coolness for those who suffer from burning pain. The antinociceptive effects of menthol appear to be mediated by the activation of kappa-opoid receptors [50]. Menthol gels can be applied frequently with little chance for side effects. Menthol can also be used as an adjunctive therapy with other transdermal medications.

Creams that contain L-arginine

The amino acid L-arginine appears to correct nitric oxide dependent endothelial dysfunction of the vasonevorum in metabolically induced neuro-ischemia. The role of nitric oxide (NO) and its NO-synthethase are well documented in the evolution of diabetic neuropathy. Correction of low nitric oxide in this disease state can be achieved locally by transcutaneous application of the relatively small molecule. Nitric oxide is formed from the end guanidine nitrogen atom of arginine. The conversion is performed by NO-synthetase. Several over the counter preparations exist (eg, Diabetiderm). L-arginine cream is particularly helpful for those neuropathic patients who complain of extremity coolness accompanied with paresthesias because the cream induces a pleasant warming sensation [45].

Prescription topicals

5% Doxepin cream (Zonalon)

Doxepin is a tricyclic norepinephrine reuptake inhibitor that has also been found to be a potent histamine blocker. Histamine is a trigger for surface skin pain fibers through the activation of H1 receptors. Blocking these receptors on peripheral neurons can be effective for treating diabetic neuropathy pain. Application is two to three times daily to the affected area. Caution should be used by patients who take monoamine oxidize inhibitors. Doxepin is particularly helpful for the elderly who cannot tolerate the anti- cholinergic effects of tricyclics taken orally, or those suffering from glaucoma [51].

5% Lidocaine patch (Lidoderm)

A membrane stabilizer and sodium channel blocker, the 5% lidocaine patch is a local anesthetic that provides relief of peripheral pain in afferent nerves. Small nociceptor C fibers have reduced frequency and amplitude, or have entirely eliminated action potentials through the blockade of sodium influx. The application of the gel or patch delivery system is applied topically by itself or in combination with other pharmacologically active agents such as prilocaine. The effects are usually limited with regard to time, and frequent applications have rarely been known to cause some minor skin irritation [26].

Isosorbide dinitrate spray (Isocard)

Isosorbide dinitrate spray, a potent local vasodilator, is a nitric oxide donator. Impaired or reduced endoneurial nitric oxide synthethase has been implicated in the pathogenesis of painful neuropathies such as those found in diabetes [52]. Yuen and colleagues [53] have demonstrated a 50% reduction of painful burning sensations recalcitrant to other therapies in a small, well-controlled study. Vasodilator therapy has been shown to promote vasonervorum angioneogenesis in diabetic rats [54]. Isosorbide dinitrate 30 mg per application can provide relief for a 24-hour period. Possible side effects include palpitations, headaches, and faintness. A glyceryl trinitrate patch can be used as an alternative if Isocard spray is not available or cannot be produced by a local compounding pharmacist [55].

Compounded transdermal gels

In recent years, centrally active pain inhibitors have serendipitously proven to be extremely effective peripherally. Through enhanced electron microscopy, spectrometry, and biochemical assays, the physiology of peripheral nerve function and receptors has been greatly elucidated. At times empiric and at other times prospective, the application of various drug classes topically can provide relief of peripheral neuropathic pain when systemic or mechanical therapies fail or are simply impractical. Sodium and calcium channels, glutamate, GABA and opioid receptors, inhibition of reuptake of neurotransmitters, can all be modulated to attenuate peripheral nerve pain. A variety of carrier molecules or delivery bases are used such as methylcellulose, 2-deoxyglucose, vanapen, lipoderm, and pluronic lecithin organogel (PLO) [48].

One of the authors (D.F.) has extensive experience using a particular formula that was created specifically to block the transmission of pain at several pathways. This peripheral nerve cream is composed of: ketamine 5%, mexiletine 2%, phenytoin 5%, clonidine 0.2%, and menthol 0.25% in a PLO gel. Naturally, many other combinations have been formulated, and they are recorded in journal articles and research papers. Below is a description of the ingredients and their activities.

Ketamine

The potent noncompetitive N-Methyl-D-Aspartate antagonist inhibits the neuronal synthesis of L-glutamate. It inhibits sympathetically maintained pain and 5-HT receptors as well as sodium channels. It has long been used for pain management in oral and intravenous forms, and has also been used transcutaneously for neuropathic and migraine pain control [56].

Mexiletine

A local anesthetic type antiarrhythmic agent, this neuronal membrane stabilizer inhibits sodium channels resulting in decreased rate and amplitude of nerve action potentials. It increases the nerve refractory periods. Found to be occasionally effective for pain management orally, its topical application has been as effective as lidocaine but with fewer side effects [57].

Phenytoin

This antiseizure drug elevates the threshold for depolarization in the resting nerve cell membrane. It thus reduces afferent nerve cell hyperexcitability in neurogenic pain syndromes. Its effect is mediated by neuronal cell membrane sodium channels. Phenytoin has been used for the treatment of painful diabetic neuropathy among other neuropathic pain states [58].

Clonidine

Originally formulated as a nasal decongestant in the 1960s, Clonidine's antihypertensive qualities made it attractive for the treatment of high blood pressure. A versatile drug, it has been shown to be effective for the treatment of a number of refractory pain syndromes including cancer pain. Administration can be sublingual, intravenous, epidural, oral, and topical. Clonidine is an alpha2 receptor agonist of the peripheral nerves. It blocks the conduction of C and A delta fibers. It inhibits the vascular smooth muscle peripherally, and increases neuronal blood flow [59].

Menthol

Menthol's ability as a neuronal calcium channel blocker and peripheral kappa opiod receptor activator has been previously described [50].

The above ingredients (Ketamine, Mexilitine, Phenytoin, Clonidine and Menthol), are mixed with a pluronic lecithin organogel to be applied topically to the affected areas three times daily. The patient is given a prescription that stipulates the appropriate percentages and is directed to a local compounding pharmacist. It can be dispensed in tubes or handy syringe dispensers in quantities of 30 to 60 mL.

Other ingredients have been used to manufacture other compounds including gabapentin, baclofen, phentolamine, dextromethorphan, amantadine, orphenadrine, guanethidine, cox II inhibitors, tricyclic antidepressants, calcium channel blockers, and other NMDA blockers, to name a few. Recently the United Kingdom has approved a tetrahyrocannabanol glossopharyngeal spray for the control of refractory neurogenic pain. Other controlled substances, such as phencyclidine and Botox, may prove useful in the future. New drug classes, such as highly specific neuronal calcium channel blockers (eg, ziconotide [Prialt]) may also some day prove useful if an appropriate transdermal carrier can be found.

The benefits of direct application of pharmacologically active substrates to target tissues with bypass of metabolism and little chance for end-organ damage and drug interactions make topical therapies safe and potentially effective primary or secondary treatment for peripheral neuropathy. Topical therapies should be considered in all cases where systemic treatment is not practical or only partially effective. A local compounding pharmacist can be an invaluable resource for the treatment of many neurogenic pain syndromes.

Physical modalities

Although several advances have occurred in the understanding and use of pharmacological agents for treatment of neuropathic pain, dangerous or debilitating side effects, costs, and drug interactions have left many physicians and patients searching for other options. One of the most studied conservative physical modalities has been the application of monochromatic infrared energy [60].

The Anodyne Therapy System (ATS) (Figs. 1, 2) produces monochromatic infrared energy (MIRE) through therapy arrays; each contains 60

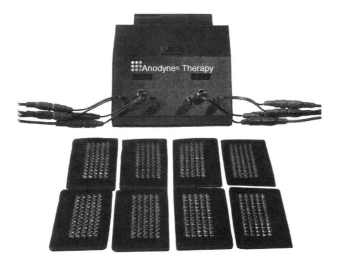

Fig. 1. Anodyne unit. (Courtesy of Anodyne Therapy, LLC, Tampa, FL.)

superluminous diodes. These diodes produce an 890 nanometer, near infra-red wavelength radiation, and are attached to a control unit that pulses the MIRE at 292 times per second [61]. A typical treatment involves placing the arrays in direct contact with the skin along the symptomatic extremities for 30–40 minutes, 3 to 7 times per week. If a wound is present, a clear plastic bag or similar barrier can be used to avoid contamination of the wound or array.

Several recent studies of ATS have demonstrated improvement in sensation and discomfort in patients who have DPN [62–64]. Leonard and

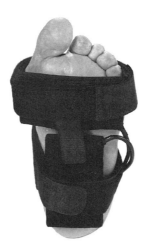

Fig. 2. Anodyne applied to the foot. (Courtesy of Anodyne Therapy, LLC, Tampa, FL.)

colleagues [63] recently reported encouraging results from a double-blind, randomized, placebo-controlled study to determine whether treatments with ATS could decrease pain or improve sensation diminished because of DPN. Significant results were shown only in the 18 patients who had less severe sensory impairments (those that could sense a 6.65 Semmes Weinstein monofilament, but were insensitive to the 5.07 monofilament at baseline). These patients reported significant improvement in sensation, improved balance, and reduced pain. The nine patients who had greater sensory impairment (measured by insensitivity to a 6.65 Semmes Weinstein monofilament) did not show statistically significant improvement [63].

DeLellis and coworkers [65] recently reported a retrospective study of 1047 subjects who had peripheral neuropathy and were treated with MIRE. They found that this treatment was associated with improved foot sensation when measured by sensitivity to a 5.07 Semmes-Weinstein monofilament. The mean number of sites insensitive to the monofilament (bilaterally; maximum or 10 sites for both feet) was 7.9 before treatment and 2.3 after treatment ($P < .0001$). In this study group, 790 subjects had DPN and the remaining 257 subjects had peripheral neuropathy with a different

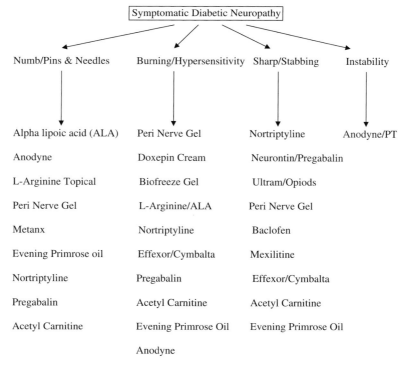

Fig. 3. Suggested treatment algorithm for symptomatic diabetic neuropathy.

etiology. Unfortunately, a report of how these two separate groups performed was not included in this review.

Although MIRE therapy seems to provide an optimistic option for non-invasive treatment of neuropathy, several features of this treatment are still not well understood. The mechanism of action, optimal dose regimen, and why some individuals don't respond to therapy are still characteristics that have not been definitively answered. Two of the authors (D.F. and B.B.) have witnessed improvement in their patients' pain and sensation with this modality, but it has always been temporary. Once therapy is stopped the symptoms return. A maintenance regimen that seems to work includes a MIRE treatment 1–2 times per week indefinitely; however, to our knowledge this has not been well studied. Fortunately, a MIRE home unit is available and is often covered by insurance. Other studied applications of MIRE include wound healing, proprioception and fall prevention, musculoskeletal pain, and edema control [62,63,66,67]. Other physical modalities such as magnet shoe insole therapy [68] have shown some benefit in reduction of neuropathy symptoms, but additional non-biased studies are needed.

A more invasive physical modality involves a surgical nerve decompression procedure and has garnered significant interest over the past several years. Outcome reports on this procedure are very encouraging and the beneficial effects seem to be permanent [69,70].

Summary

Although numerous modalities are now available for the treatment of peripheral neuropathy, it can be difficult to find an effective treatment for each particular patient. Fig. 3 shows a suggested treatment algorithm. The intention of this algorithm is not to create a recipe to follow for every situation. Consultation with a pain specialist, neurologist, or peripheral nerve surgeon who has knowledge and training in the latest neuropathy treatments is prudent for cases that are recalcitrant to standard care. Many effective non-prescription and safe prescription modalities exist that can greatly improve the symptoms of patients who suffer from peripheral neuropathy.

References

[1] Carter GT, Galer BS. Advances in the management of neuropathic pain. Phys Med Rehabil Clin N Am 2001;12:447–59.

[2] Dyck PJ, Kratz KM, Karnes JL, et al. The prevalence by staged severity of various types of diabetic neuropathy, retinopathy, and nephropathy in a population-based cohort. Neurology 1993;43:817–24.

[3] Brooks PJ, Francisco GE. Drug therapy of diabetic neuropathy. Clin Pod Med Surg 1992; 9(2):257–74.

[4] Armstrong DG, Lavery LA, Harkless LB. Validation of a diabetic wound classification system: the contribution of depth, infection, and ischemia to risk of amputation. Diabetes Care 1998;21:855–9.

[5] Low P, Dotson R. Symptom treatment of painful neuropathy. JAMA 1998;280:1863–4.

[6] National diabetes fact sheet, 2005. Available at: http://www.diabetes.org/uedocuments/NationalDiabetesFactSheetRev.pdf. Accessed May 2005.

[7] Misha-Miroslav B, Serra J. Pharmacologic management part I: better-studied neuropathic pain diseases. Pain Med 2004;5(S1):S28–47.

[8] Podwall D, Gooch C. Diabetic neuropathy: clinical features, etiology and therapy. Curr Neurol Neurosci Rep 2004;4:55–61.

[9] Shaw JE, Zimmet PZ. The epidemiology of diabetic neuropathy. Diabetes Rev 1999;7: 245–52.

[10] Maizels M, McCarberg B. Antidepressants and antiepileptic drugs for chronic non-cancer pain. Am Fam Physician 2005;71(3):483–90.

[11] Sindrup SH, Bach FW, Madsen C, et al. Venlafaxine versus imipramine in painful polyneuropathy: a randomized, controlled trial. Neurology 2003;60:1284–9.

[12] Watson CP, Vernich L, Chipman M, et al. Nortriptyline versus amitriptyline in postherpetic neuralgia: a randomized trial. Neurology 1998;51(4):1166–71.

[13] Goldstein DJ, Lu Y, Iyengar S, et al. Duloxetine in the treatment of the pain associated with diabetic neuropathy. Presented at the 156th Annual Meeting of the American Psychiatric Association. SanFrancisco, May 17–22, 2003.

[14] Wernicke JF, Lu Y, D'Souza DN, et al. Duloxetine at doses of 60 mgQD and 60 mg BID is effective treatment of diabetic neuropathic pain. Presented at the 56th Annual meeting of the American Academy of Neurology. SanFrancisco, April 24–May 1, 2004.

[15] Wernicke JF, Rosen A, Lu Y, et al. The safety of Duloxetine in the long-term treatment of diabetic neuropathic pain. Presented at the 23rd Annual Scientific Meeting of the American Pain Society. Vancouver, May 6–9, 2004.

[16] Bymaster FP, Dreshfield-Ahmad LJ, Threlkeld PG, et al. Comparative affinity of duloxetine and venlafaxine for serotonin and norepinephrine transporters in vitro and in vivo, human serotonin receptor subtypes, and other neuronal receptors. Neuropsychopharmacol 2001; 25(6):871–80.

[17] Waitekus AB, Kirkpatrick P. Duloxetine hydrocloride. Nat Rev Drug Discov 2004;3(11): 907–8.

[18] Rosenstock J, Tuchman M, LaMoreaux L, et al. Pregabalin for the treatment of diabetic peripheral neuropathy: a double –blind, placebo-controlled trial. Pain 2004;110(3): 628–38.

[19] Sharma U, Allen R, Glessner C, et al. Pregabalin effectively relieves pain in patients with diabetic peripheral neuropathy. Diabetes 2000;49(Suppl 1):A167.

[20] Lesser H, Sharma U, LaMoreaux L, et al. Pregabalin relieves symptoms of painful diabetic neuropathy: a randomized controlled trial. Neurology 2004;63(11):2104–10.

[21] Dworkin RH, Corbin AE, Young JP, et al. Pregabalin for the treatment of postherpetic neuralgia: a randomized, placebo-controlled trial. Neurology 2003;60:1274–83.

[22] Sabatowski R, Galvez R, Cherry DA. Pregabalin reduces pain and improves sleep and mood disturbance in patients with post-herpetic neuralgia: results of a randomized, placebo-controlled clinical trial. Pain 2004;109:26–35.

[23] Weiner RS, editor. Pain management: a practical guide for clinicians. 6th edition. Boca Raton (FL): CRC Press; 2002.

[24] Duhmke RM, Cornblath DD, Hollingshead JR. Tramadol for neuropathic pain. Cochrane Database Syst Rev 2004;(2):CD003726.

[25] Sindrup SH, Andersen G, Madsen C, et al. Tramadol relieves pain and allodynia in polyneuropathy: a randomized, double-blind, contolled trial. Pain 1999;83(1):85–90.

[26] Barbano RL, Herrmann DN, Hart-Gouleau S, et al. Effectiveness, tolerability, and impact on quality of life of the 5% lidocaine patch in diabetic polyneuropathy. Arch Neurol 2004;(June):914–8.

[27] Lidoderm prescribing information. Chadds Ford (PA): Endo Pharmaceuticals Inc; 2004. Available at: www.lidoderm.com/safety.aspx. Accessed April, 2005.

[28] Jamal GA. The use of gamma linolenic acid in the prevention and treatment of diabetic neuropathy. Diabet Med 1994;11(2):145–9.

[29] Ford I, Cotter MA, Cameron NE, et al. The effects of treatment with alpha-lipoic acid or evening primrose oil on vascular hemostatic and lipid risk factors, blood flow, and peripheral nerve conduction in the streptozotocin-diabetic rat. Metabolism 2001;50(8):868–75.

[30] Anonymous. Acetyl-L-carnitine [letter]. Altern Med Rev 1999;4(6):438–41.

[31] De Grandis D, Minardi C. Acetyl-L-carnitine (levacecarnine) in the treatment of diabetic neuropathy. A long-term, randomized, double-blind, placebo-controlled study. Drugs R D 2002;3(4):223–31.

[32] Sima AA, Calvani M, Mehra M, et al. Acetyl-L-carnitine improves pain, nerve regeneration, and vibratory perception in patients with chronic diabetic neuropathy: an analysis of two randomized placebo-controlled trials. Diabetes Care 2005;28(1):89–94.

[33] Nicklander KK, McPheee BR, Low PA, et al. Alpha-lipoic acid: antioxidant potency against lipid peroxidation of neural tissues in vitro and implications for diabetic neuropathy. Free Radic Biol Med 1996;21(5):631–9.

[34] Packer L, Kraemer K, Rimbach G. Molecular aspects of lipoic acid in the prevention of diabetes complications. Nutrition 2001;17(10):888–95.

[35] Ametov AS, Barinov A, Dyck PJ, et al. The sensory symptoms of diabetic polyneuropathy are improved with alpha-lipoic acid: the SYDNEY trial. Diabetes Care 2003;26(3):770–6.

[36] Reljanovic M, Reichel G, Rett K, et al. Treatment of diabetic polyneuropathy with the antioxidant thioctic acid (alpha-lipoic acid): a two year multicenter randomized double blind placebo-controlled trial (ALADIN II). Alpha Lipoic Acid in Diabetic Neuropathy. Free Radic Res 1999;31(3):171–9.

[37] Obrosova IG, Fathallah L, Stevens MJ. Taurine counteracts oxidative stress and nerve growth factor deficit in early experimental diabetic neuropathy. Exp Neurol 2001;172(1): 211–9.

[38] Li F, Obrosova IG, Abatan O, et al. Taurine replacement attenuates hyperalgesia and abnormal calcium signaling in sensory neurons of STZ-D rats. Am J Physiol Endocrinol Metab 2005;288(1):E29–36.

[39] Ambrosch A, Dierkes J, Lobmann R, et al. Relation between homocysteinaemia and diabetic neuropathy in patients with Type 2 diabetes mellitus. Diabet Med 2001;18:185–92.

[40] Willems FF, et al. Pharmocokinetic study on the utilisation of 5-methyltetrahudrofolate and folic acid in patients with coronary artery disease. BMJ 2004;141:825–30.

[41] Mauskop A, Altura BM. Role of magnesium in the pathogenesis and treatment of migraines. Clin Neurosci 1998;5(1):24–7.

[42] Sima AA, Dunlap J, Davidson E, et al. Supplemental myo-inositol prevents L-fucose induced diabetic neuropathy. Diabetes 1997;46(2):306.

[43] Olin VI, Belikova TV, Pushkova ES. Diabetes mellitus in the elderly: succinic acid compounds in treating diabetic neuropathies. Adv Gerontol 2002;9:83–7 [in Russian].

[44] Yorek MA, Coppey LJ, Gellett JS, et al. Effect of treatment of diabetic rats with dehydroepiandrosterone on vascular and neural function. Am J Physiol Endocrinol Metab 2002; 283(5):E1067–75.

[45] Witte MB, Barbul A. Role of nitric oxide in wound repair. Am J Surg 2002;183(4):406–12.

[46] Stracke H, Hammes HP, Werkmann D, et al. Efficacy of benfotiamine versus thiamine on function and glycation products of peripheral nerves in diabetic rats. Exp Clin Endocrinol Diabetes 2001;109(6):330–6.

[47] Haupt E, Ledermann H, Kopcke W. Benfotiamine in the treatment of diabetic poly neuropathy—a three-week randomized, controlled pilot study (BEDIP study). Int J Clin Pharmacol Ther 2005;43(2):71–7.

[48] Transdermal gel pain management. Available at: http://www.pinepharmacy.com/pain_management_md.asp#gel. Accessed April 21, 2005.

[49] DeLee JC, Drez D, Miller MD. Orthopedic sports medicine. 2nd edition. Vol. 1. Philadelphia: W.B. Saunders; 2002. p. 452–4.

[50] Galeotti N. Menthol: a natural analgesic compound. Neurosci Lett 2002;322(3):145–8.

[51] McCleane G. Doxepin hydrochloride, capsaicin and a combination of both produces analgesia in chronic human neuropathic pain: double-blind, placebo-controlled study. Br J Pharmacol 2000;49(6):574–9.

[52] Pitei DL, Watkins PJ, Edmonds ME. No-dependent smooth muscle vasodilation is reduced in NIDDM patients with peripheral sensory neuropathy. Diabet Med 1997;14:284–90.

[53] Yuen KCJ, Baker NR, Rayman G. Treatment of chronic painful diabetic neuropathy with isosorbide dinitrate spray. Diabetes Care 2002;25(10):1699–703.

[54] Cameron NE, Cotter MA, Ferguson K, et al. Angiotensin converting enzyme inhibition prevents the development of muscle and nerve dysfunction and stimulates angiogenesis in streptozotocin-diabetic rats. Diabetologia 1992;35:12–8 [abstract].

[55] Rayman G, Baker NR, Krishnan ST. Glyceryl trinitrate patches as an alternative to isosorbide dinitrate spray in the treatment of chronic painful diabetic neuropathy. Diabetes Care 2003;26(9):2697–8.

[56] Lynch ME, Clark AJ, Sawynok J. A pilot study examining topical amytriptylene, ketamine, and a combination of both in treatment of neuropathic pain. Clin J Pain 2003;19:323–8.

[57] Milch RA. Neuropathic pain: implications for the surgeon. Surg Clin N Am 2005;85(2): 225–36.

[58] Pray WS. Consult your pharmacist-shingles: a rising threat with age. US Pharmacist 1997; 22(8).

[59] Clonidine hydrochloride. Mosby's Drug Consult [Password protected]. Available at: http://home.mdconsult.com/das/drug/body/367875243/1/846.html. Accessed May 17, 2005.

[60] Goldberg N. Monochromatic infrared photo energy and DPN Diab. Microvasc Complications Today 2005;March/April:30–2.

[61] Burke TJ. Questions and answers about MIRE treatment. Adv Skin Wound Care 2003;16: 369–71.

[62] Kochman AB, Carnegie DH, Burke TJ. Symptomatic reversal of peripheral neuropathy in patients with diabetes. JAPMA 2002;92:125.

[63] Leonard DR, Farooqi HM, Myers S. Restoration of sensation, reduced pain, and improved balance in subjects with diabetic peripheral neuropathy. Diabetes Care 2004;27:168–72.

[64] Prendergast JJ, Miranda G, Sanchez M. Reduced sensory impairment in patients with peripheral neuropathy. Endocr Pract 2004;10:24–30.

[65] DeLellis SL, Carnegie DH, Burke TJ. Improved sensitivity in patients with peripheral neuropathy effects of monochromatic infrared photo energy. JAPMA 2005;95(2):143–7.

[66] Horwitz LR, Burke TJ, Carnegie D. Augmentation of wound healing using monochromatic infrared energy exploration of a new technology for wound management. Adv Wound Care 1999;12:35–40.

[67] Thomasson TL. Effects of skin-contact monochromatic infrared irradiation on tendonitis, capsulitis, and myofascial pain. J Neuro Orthop Med Surg 1996;16:242–5.

[68] Weintraub MI. Magnetic bio-stimulation in painful diabetic peripheral neuropathy: an novel intervention a randomized, double-placebo, crossover study. Am J Pain Managet 1999;9:8–17.

[69] Biddinger KR, Amend MA. The role of surgical decompression for diabetic neuropathy. Foot Ankle Clin N Am 2004;9:239–54.

[70] Dellon AL. Diabetic neuropathy: review of a surgical approach to restore sensation, relieve pain, and prevent ulceration and amputation. Foot Ankle Int 2004;25(10):749–55.

ELSEVIER
SAUNDERS

Clin Podiatr Med Surg
23 (2006) 531–543

CLINICS IN
PODIATRIC
MEDICINE AND
SURGERY

Electromyography and Nerve Conduction Studies of the Lower Extremity: Uses and Limitations

William G. Buxton, MD*, Justin E. Dominick, MD

*UCLA-Santa Monica Neurologic Associates, 1245 16th Street, Suite 309,
Santa Monica, CA 90404, USA*

Although commonly referred to as an EMG, a complete electrodiagnostic study (EDX) involves nerve conduction studies (NCS) and electromyography (EMG). The two complement each other, in that both give information about peripheral nerves and muscles. Each in isolation does not yield a complete assessment of the cause of the symptoms being assessed in a limb or limbs.

In nerve conduction studies, a small amount of electrical current—1–100 mA—is applied to the skin over a peripheral nerve for 0.05–1 millisecond. In motor nerve conduction studies, the elicited compound motor action potential is recorded from a muscle innervated by the nerve, usually with surface electrodes. In sensory nerve conduction studies, the response is recorded over the nerve itself. Marked slowing of the response is generally indicative of demyelination along the nerve being assessed. A decrease in amplitude can occur because of axonal loss or myopathy, which can be further distinguished by needle electromyography. Additional testing commonly performed includes the H-reflex, produced through activation of a monosynaptic reflex arc, and F-waves, which increase the sensitivity for segmental demyelination along the course of an entire nerve [1].

In the second portion of the neurodiagnostic assessment, needle electromyography, a narrow (26–27 gauge) needle electrode is inserted into the belly of the muscle being investigated while the patient voluntarily contracts the muscle. The real-time potential between the electrode on the needle's tip and another electrode, usually on the surface, is recorded. This is amplified and digitized on a monitor, which provides a representation of the

---

* Corresponding author.
E-mail address: wbuxton@ucla.edu (W.G. Buxton).

summated action potentials generated in individual muscle fibers when a motor unit (anterior horn cell in the spinal cord and all of its innervated muscle fibers) fires [2]. Based on the morphology of the units and their firing pattern, the examiner can determine whether a neurogenic (e.g. axonal loss vs. demyelination) or myopathic process is at hand, and, especially in the case of axonal loss, how long the process has been present. The patient then relaxes the muscle, and the examiner observes for spontaneous activity at rest, such as fibrillations, which usually indicate active denervation, but can also be seen in some myopathies [3].

For neurogenic processes, the timing of the exam is important. In the first 1–2 weeks after a neurogenic injury, the only abnormality that may be seen on neurodiagnostic testing is a decrease in recruitment on EMG, a change in the firing pattern of motor neurons. However, such changes are usually very limited if present at all [4]. Therefore, the usefulness of neurodiagnostic testing increases significantly 3 weeks after symptom onset, when fibrillation potentials begin to appear [5].

Based upon the types of deficits present in the complete NCS and EMG, symptoms in a limb can be characterized as neurogenic (ie, caused by nerve dysfunction) or myopathic. In the case of a neurogenic process, the pattern of affected nerves and muscles facilitates localization of a lesion, whether in a single nerve (mononeuropathy), a spinal root (radiculopathy), plexus (plexopathy), or nerves as a whole (polyneuropathy).

This article focuses on common neurogenic processes that cause foot pain and numbness, specifically polyneuropathy, lumbosacral radiculopathy, and mononeuropathies of the peroneal and plantar nerves. Brief mention is made of sciatic mononeuropathy and lumbosacral plexopathies. For each, there is an assessment of the usefulness and limitations of neurodiagnostic testing for diagnosis as well as a brief description of each of the clinical syndromes.

Lumbosacral radiculopathy

Lumbosacral radiculopathy can result in foot discomfort, such as numbness or dysesthetic pain. However, it does not usually cause local foot pain [6]. It results from any process that causes loss of axons or myelin in the spinal nerve roots as they pass through the intervertebral foramina. The process can be structural, such as from disc bulge or spondylosis; ischemic, as is common in patients who have diabetes; inflammatory, as in Guillian-Barre Syndrome, or Acute Inflammatory Demyelinating Polyradiculoneuropahy; or infiltrative, as in infection or malignancy, among others. Transection can also cause radiculopathy [5,7]. Patients may experience foot discomfort, such as sensory loss or burning in the affected dermatome. Patients who have lumbosacral radiculopathy usually experience pain in a radicular pattern. Frequent descriptors of the pain include jabbing, sharp, or lancinating. Most patients report a history of previous back pain, generally aching and deep. However, isolated radicular pain does occur [8]. The sensory and motor findings found in each lumbosacral level are included in Table 1 [9].

Neurodiagnostic testing can be very helpful in the assessment of whether pain is radicular in nature. The needle EMG identifies denervation and re-innervation in affected muscles. Localizing changes to a given myotome with normal sensory responses supports a diagnosis of radiculopathy, especially if there is paraspinal muscle involvement. The presence of spontaneous activity at rest indicates active denervation. Reports of the sensitivity of needle EMG for radiculopathy vary; Linden and Berlit [10] report a little less than 80%. The addition of H-reflexes of the gastrocnemius and tibialis anterior increased sensitivity to around 90% [10].

There are numerous advantages of neurodiagnostic testing for the assessment of lumbosacral radiculopathy. If there is no structural component to a root lesion, such as in inflammatory processes, it may be the only objective test that is abnormal. Although many aspects of the EDX are dependent on patient effort, many are not, which facilitates objective testing if patient effort is limited volitionally or by other medical problems, such as upper motor neuron dysfunction. It can also distinguish more distal processes, such as

Table 1
Symptoms and signs association with lumbar radiculopathy

Root	Pain distribution	Dermatomal sensory distribution	Weakness	Affected reflex
L1	Inguinal region	Inguinal region	Hip flexion	Cremasteric
L2	Inguinal region and anterior thigh	Anterior thigh	Hip flexion, hip adduction	Cremasteric, thigh adductor
L3	Anterior thigh and knee	Distal anteromedial thigh including knee	Knee extension, hip flexion, hip adduction	Patellar, thigh adductor
L4	Anterior thigh, medial aspect leg	Medial leg	Knee extension, hip flexion, hip adduction	Patellar
L5	Posterolateral thigh, lateral leg, medial foot	Lateral leg, dorsal foot, and great toe	Dorsiflexion foot/toes, knee flexion hip extension[a]	—
S1	Posterior thigh and leg, and lateral foot	Posterolateral leg and lateral aspect of foot	Plantar flexion foot/toes, knee flexion, hip extension[a]	Achilles

[a] Most specific.

From Deveraux, M. Neck and low back pain. Med Clin N Am 2003;87:643–62; with permission.

plexopathies, that can clinically resemble radiculopathy. Finally, in the hands of experienced examiners, neurodiagnostic evaluations have a very low false-positive rate [4]. A thorough assessment of proximal and distal muscles innervated by L5 and S1 can be very instructive for finding the presence of radiculopathy at those levels in someone who has distal denervation from polyneuropathy, a very common combination [4]. This is helpful because it is common for lumbar imaging to result in incidental findings of little or no clinical significance, especially in individuals who are middle-age or older. One study reported disc bulges in just over half of a pool of asymptomatic individuals without back pain [11].

There are limitations, however, and timing is important. Even in established, mild lumbar radiculopathies, the study is not entirely 100% sensitive. Although neurodiagnostic testing establishes whether denervation or reinnervation is present and localizes such processes, it does not address etiology, whether structural or nonstructural. Particularly in the lumbar spine, it does not localize whether a compressive lesion is within the central spinal canal or in the neural foramen. Also, there can be considerable overlap between the findings of radiculopathy with other causes of denervation, such as polyneuropathy [4]. Finally, it is essential to sample multiple limb muscles because denervation has been found in the paraspinal muscles of up to 14% of asymptomatic individuals [4,12].

Polyneuropathy

Polyneuropathies usually begin with a sense of numbness in the feet. There may be associated burning, tingling, or sometimes an alteration of sensation. Many describe a feeling of walking on gravel or rocks. More pronounced alteration in sensation may result in allodynia, the perception of painless stimulation as painful. The onset is usually slow but isn't universally so. The findings are usually symmetrical. If there is large-fiber involvement, imbalance may be a predominant symptom. Clues on physical exam include decreased sensation to temperature, vibration, or very light touch with a cotton wisp in a stocking distribution, and there is frequently distal loss in the upper extremities. Deep tendon reflexes are usually decreased, especially at the ankles. If there is very mild large-fiber involvement, the only abnormality on exam may be a positive Romberg test. If there is motor involvement, atrophy or weakness of intrinsic foot muscles may be present. Autonomic involvement may also be present, particularly in neuropathies caused by diabetes and amyloidosis [13,14].

A patient's medical history can indicate risk for polyneuropathy. Worldwide, leprosy is the predominant treatable cause. In the developed world, diabetes mellitus and alcohol use are the most common etiologies [15]. Pain is associated with some polyneuropathies: amyloidosis, diabetes mellitus, some hereditary neuropathies, and vasculitic neuropathies. Infectious neuropathies (particularly Lyme disease and human immunodeficiency virus) are frequently painful, and pain has also been reported with metabolic neuropathies, such as those associated with uremia or thyroid dysfunction. Finally, many toxic polyneuropathies are associated with pain [15,16]. Polyneuropathies in which pain is a predominant or associated symptom are found in Tables 2 and 3, along with associated diagnostic studies [15]. In addition to amyloidosis, other paraproteinemias, including multiple myeloma, are associated with polyneuropathies. Furthermore, the combination of a monoclonal protein with polyneuropathy, but no evidence of any underlying disorder, is quite common, and constitutes monoclonal gammopathy of uncertain significance.

Electrodiagnostic testing can be very helpful in the diagnosis of sensory polyneuropathy. In nerve conduction testing, the patterns of abnormalities distinguish between axonal and demyelinating processes, which can help to ascertain etiologies, particularly in the case of acute demyelinating inflammatory polyneuropathy [15], which can progress rapidly to include bulbar and autonomic processes. If a patient has only motor or sensory symptoms, the combination of nerve conduction studies and needle EMG frequently reveals mild subclinical abnormalities of the other. In the case of bilateral lower lumbar and sacral radicular disease (which when mild can resemble a sensory polyneuropathy), the involvement of proximal L5 and S1 innervated muscles on EMG with normal sensory responses can lead a clinician more toward a diagnosis of radiculopathy, because radiculopathies yield normal sensory responses (see section on lumbosacral radiculopathy).

Table 2
Primary painful polyneuropathies

Polyneuropathies	Diagnosis
Idiopathic	
Idiopathic distal small fiber neuropathy[a]	
Inflammatory	
Vasculitic neuropathy	Vasculitic workup/biopsy
Perineuritis	Biopsy
Hereditary	
Fabry[a] disease	Alpha-galactosidase A
HSAN type V	
Tangier disease[a]	Hypocholesterolemia, low serum alpha-lipoprotein
Metabolic	
Amyloidosis[a]	Biopsy/genetic testing
Diabetes[a]	AM glucose/2 hour GTT
Painfull symmetrical polyneuropathy	
Asymmetric polyradiculoneuropathy	
Truncal mononeuropathy	

[a] Denotes small fiber neuropathy.

From Wein TH, Albers JW. Electrodiagnostic approach to the patient with suspected peripheral polyneuropathy. Neurol Clin N Am 2002;20:503–26; with permission.

Table 3
Polyneuropathies associated with pain

Polyneuropathies	Diagnosis
Idiopathic	
Cryotogenic sensory neuropathy	Skin biopsy PGP 9.5 stain
Infectious	
HIV	HIV serology
Inflammatory	
AIDP	
Malignancies	
Paraneoplastic	
Small cell carcinoma	CT chest
Lymphoma	Bone marrow
Other carcinomas	Malignancy workup
Paraproteinemia	Protein electrophoresis
Multiple myeloma	Bence-Jones proteins
Waldenstrom	Bone marrow
Metabolic	
Hypothyroidism	TSH
Uremia	BUN, creatinine
Nutritional	
Alcohol	History
B12/thiamine deficiency	B12/folate
Toxic	
Arsenic/thallium	Mees' lines
Dideoxyinosine	EMG/history
Dideoxycytosine	EMG/history
Isoniazid/pyridoxine deficiency	EMG/history
Nitrofurantoin	EMG/history
n-Hexane	EMG/history/biopsy
Vincristine	EMG/history

From Wein TH, Albers JW. Electrodiagnostic approach to the patient with suspected peripheral polyneuropathy. Neurol Clin N Am 2002;20:503–26; with permission.

Therefore, neurodiagnostic testing can help to distinguish polyneuropathy from other causes of foot pain and numbness. The main limitation lies in the observation that 23% of poluneuropathies are idiopathic small fiber neuropathy [17], and nerve conduction studies are not particularly sensitive for small fiber polyneuropathies. Using the sural sensory nerve action potential amplitude, Wolfe and colleagues [18] reported a sensitivity of 69%. Using additional distal indices, their sensitivity increased to 77%. The ratio of the sural and radial sensory potential amplitudes has been found to be abnormal in 51% of diabetic patients, many without clinical symptoms of polyneuropathy, compared with 29.3% for the absolute sural sensory amplitude. Assessment of F-waves in electrodiagnostic testing of patients with diabetes mellitus has been shown to yield a higher percentage of abnormal findings as compared to routine sensory testing alone [19]. If an assessment of the dorsal branch of the sural nerve is added to that of the sural nerve, nerve conduction testing increased in sensitivity from 77% to 97% [20].

Likewise, Kushnir and colleagues [21] found low amplitudes or abnormal conduction in 49% and 57% respectively when they added an investigation of the medial dorsal superficial peroneal nerve to their routine sural assessment. Finally, a needle EMG examination can help identify subtle, subclinical motor involvement, particularly if intrinsic foot muscles are sampled [17].

Tarsal tunnel syndrome

Tarsal tunnel syndrome (sometimes referred to as medial or posterior tarsal tunnel syndrome, to distinguish it from anterior tarsal tunnel syndrome) is an entrapment neuropathy of the tibial nerve or one or more of its branches (medial plantar, lateral plantar, and calcaneal nerves) beneath the flexor retinaculum behind and inferior to the medial malleolus. It may be confused with a variety of other conditions, including plantar fasciitis, rheumatoid arthritis, foot strain, interdigital neuroma, sacral radiculopathy, and peripheral neuropathy, which makes it difficult to diagnose. The condition is often suspected based on history, clinical examination, and imaging findings, although electrodiagnostic studies are usually required for confirmation. Typical electrodiagnostic findings that support a diagnosis of tarsal tunnel syndrome include: delayed latencies of the medial and lateral plantar nerves across the ankle; delayed latencies or low amplitude compound muscle action potentials of the medial and lateral plantar nerves, recording at the abductor hallucis and abductor digiti minimi, respectively; and denervation of tibial nerve innervated intrinsic foot muscles [22–30]. There are several issues, however, that make electrodiagnostic confirmation of tarsal tunnel syndrome difficult.

In contrast to sensory nerve conduction studies of the upper extremity (eg, median and ulnar nerves), which are easily recordable and reproducible in normal subjects, it may be difficult to similarly record responses from the sensory nerves of the foot, in part because of their smaller amplitudes, as well as their possible absence even in normal individuals. Guiloff and Sheratt [26] studied the medial plantar sensory nerve in 69 control subjects, who ranged in age from 13 to 81 years. They stimulated the nerve with ring electrodes at the great toe and recorded at a point near the medial malleolus. Medial plantar sensory action potentials were absent in 3 of the 16 patients who were 60 years or older. Ponsford [31] studied medial and lateral plantar sensory action potentials. He stimulated the nerves in the sole and used surface electrodes at the ankle to record in 59 healthy subjects, ranging in age from 14 to 85 years. Medial plantar sensory action potentials were recordable in all of these subjects, even those over age 60. However, lateral plantar sensory action potentials were absent in 20 of 29 subjects 60 years of age or older. Despite this, an absent medial plantar response in itself is not necessarily pathologic if it is absent on the contralateral or asymptomatic side. Stimulation of the medial and lateral plantar nerves in the sole produces mixed nerve action potentials (ie, motor and sensory), although these potentials represent predominantly sensory fibers [23,32].

Guiloff and Sheratt's [26] method of stimulating at the great toe resulted in small amplitude responses, a mean of 2.3 μV, and required averaging many responses. Saeed and Gatens [32] obtained responses in only 17% of normal subjects when the medial plantar nerve was stimulated at the great toe, and in none of the subjects when the lateral plantar nerve was stimulated at the little toe. In addition, the mean amplitudes of the medial and lateral sensory action potentials were found to decrease with age [26,31]. Stimulation of these nerves in the sole, as compared with the toes, may result in relatively larger amplitude responses [31–33].

The medial calcaneal nerve is a pure sensory branch of the tibial nerve and supplies sensation to the heel. It, too, may be implicated in cases of tarsal tunnel syndrome, and is potentially amenable to electrodiagnostic study by recording at the medial aspect of the calcaneus, and stimulating the tibial nerve approximately 10 cm proximal to this. There is variation in the anatomy and course of the medial calcaneal nerve, however, which may run superficial to the flexor retinaculum [34]. In such cases, the nerve response may be normal, despite the presence of symptoms suggestive of tarsal tunnel syndrome.

It is also possible to assess the medial and lateral plantar motor fibers by stimulating the tibial nerve behind the medial malleolus above the flexor retinaculum, and by recording over the abductor hallucis and abductor digiti minimi, respectively. Tarsal tunnel syndrome may be suggested by prolonged distal motor latencies or reduced compound muscle action potential amplitudes of one or both of these nerves [23,27,29]. Normal motor responses may be found, however, and do not necessarily exclude the diagnosis of tarsal tunnel syndrome [22,25,29,30]. Abnormalities may be restricted to sensory fibers, especially early in the course and depending on the severity of entrapment, such as may occur with carpal tunnel syndrome [35]. Oh and colleagues [30] found a prolonged distal motor latency in the medial or lateral plantar nerve in only 52.4% of cases, but abnormal sensory responses were found in 90.5% of the cases. Technical factors, such as foot deformities, calloused skin, and edema about the foot or ankle, among others, may also lead to difficulties in accurately recording motor and especially sensory responses.

Needle electromyography of intrinsic foot muscles supplied by the tibial nerve may help to diagnose tarsal tunnel syndrome if there is evidence of chronic or active denervation. However, these results should be interpreted with caution. Gatens and Saaed [36] performed EMG on the feet of 70 asymptomatic subjects. Positive sharp waves were found in 10% of the abductor hallucis and in 11.4% of the abductor digiti minimi. They found fibrillations in 5.7% of the abductor digiti minimi [36]. Falck and Alaranta [37] found fibrillations or positive sharp waves in 43.4% of the abductor digiti minimi in 53 asymptomatic individuals. Possible causes for these changes may include age-related nerve degeneration and mechanical trauma to the nerves as a result of normal everyday activity [36,37]. Boon and Harper [38] found fibrillations in 21% of the abductor hallucis in normal subjects (10% in those under age 60; 30% in those over age 60) [38]. Furthermore, it may be difficult for patients to activate these muscles [38], and needle examination of the intrinsic foot muscles is quite painful.

Anterior tarsal tunnel syndrome

Anterior tarsal tunnel syndrome is another potential cause of sensory or motor symptoms in the foot in which the deep peroneal nerve is compressed or entrapped as it passes under the extensor retinaculum at the ankle [39–43]. Symptoms may consist of possible weakness or fatigue in the foot, and pain, numbness, or paresthesias in the web space between the first and second toes, ankle, or dorsum of the foot, which may radiate proximally into the leg and may be worse at night [39–43].

Electrodiagnostic techniques that may be useful in the diagnosis of anterior tarsal tunnel syndrome consist of motor nerve conduction studies of the deep peroneal nerve, recording at the extensor digitorum brevis muscle, sensory studies of the deep peroneal nerve, recording at the interspace between the first and second toes, and needle examination of the extensor digitorum brevis (EDB). The typical finding on motor nerve conduction studies is a prolonged distal latency [39,41–43]. Atrophy of the extensor digitorum brevis itself is not uncommon, in which case a prolonged distal motor latency may be seen in combination with reduced compound motor action potential amplitude. Nerves in the legs and feet may be more subject to cooling than those in the hands and arms. As such, it is always important to ensure that any prolonged latency is not caused by temperature effects. Another factor to consider is the reported prevalence of an accessory peroneal nerve in 28% of the population, in which a branch from the superficial peroneal nerve supplies the extensor digitorum brevis after passing behind the lateral malleolus [44]. In such cases, the compound motor action potential amplitude at the extensor digitorum brevis is typically smaller. Stimulation of the deep peroneal nerve is at the ankle compared with stimulation of the common peroneal nerve at the knee, which may lead to confusion if this possibility is not considered.

For sensory nerve conduction studies, one stimulates the deep peroneal nerve at the ankle, and records in the interspace between the first and second toes. Lee and coworkers [45] obtained responses in all of the 40 normal subjects they studied (21–50 years old). The average sensory nerve action potential amplitude was 3.4 μV (range 1.6–6.6 μV) [45]. Posas and coworkers [46,47] studied the deep peroneal sensory nerve in 18 asymptomatic subjects and found an average amplitude of 5.16 μV. These are small, sometimes difficult to record responses which usually require averaging. If a response is absent or abnormal on one side, it is important to study the nerve on the contralateral side for comparison. It is also important to keep in mind that responses may be absent in normal, otherwise asymptomatic individuals. This may be even more likely in older individuals, as described above in reference to the medial and lateral plantar sensory nerves. Ponsford [48] studied the deep peroneal sensory nerve orthodromically, stimulating on the dorsum of the foot between the first and second toes, and recording over the deep peroneal nerve at the ankle. He noted a significant reduction in the amplitude in asymptomatic subjects over age 40, and questioned the clinical significance of an absent response in older individuals.

Needle electromyography of the extensor digitorum brevis is often used to confirm the diagnosis of anterior tarsal tunnel syndrome by showing evidence of denervation [39,41–43]. As described above in electrodiagnosis of tarsal tunnel syndrome, interpretation of abnormalities can be difficult because denervation changes may be found in the feet of otherwise asymptomatic individuals. Falck and Alaranta [37] found fibrillations or positive sharp waves in approximately 28% of the EDB in 53 healthy subjects. Gatens and Saeed [36] found evidence of denervation, which consisted of fibrillations or positive sharp waves, in 17% of the EDB in normal subjects. Positive sharp waves were seen in the EDB in 15.7% of normal subjects studied by Wiechers [49]. Rosselle and Stevens [50] found fibrillations or positive sharp waves in the EDB of 29% of healthy subjects 20–30 years of age.

Superficial peroneal neuropathy

Another potential source of numbness, tingling, and pain in the leg, ankle, or foot is an abnormality of the superficial peroneal nerve. Several techniques for studying the superficial peroneal sensory nerve have been described [51–55]. Although a potentially useful and straightforward study, absent responses in otherwise normal individuals must be interpreted with caution, and do not necessarily indicate nerve pathology. Izzo and colleagues [51] were unable to elicit a response from the intermediate branch in 2% of healthy subjects. Levin and coworkers [53] were unable to elicit a response in 8.6% of normal subjects, and DiBenedetto [56] found no recordable responses in 2%–3% of otherwise healthy individuals. Thus, as with any abnormal or absent response, comparison with the asymptomatic limb should be made. If a response is not found on the contralateral or asymptomatic side, results should be interpreted cautiously.

Other neurogenic causes of foot pain

Finally, there are two proximal processes that warrant brief mention: sciatic neuropathy and lumbosacral plexopathy. The sciatic nerve is not uncommonly compressed from prolonged pressure, injection, or hip surgery. Fibers that will join the peroneal nerve when the sciatic nerve splits into tibial and peroneal divisions are more susceptible to injury. As a result, a sciatic neuropathy can often mimic a peroneal mononeuropathy. The only overt sensory involvement may be over the lateral aspect of the foot and shin. Pain can be marked. A foot drop is usually present. However, if the motor involvement is mild, neurodiagnostic testing can reveal subtle changes in extra-peroneal muscles, localizing the process to the sciatic nerve. Abnormalites of sensory potentials and normal paraspinal muscles would distinguish a sciatic neuropathy from a lumbar radiculopathy [57].

Similarly, a lesion of the lumbosacral trunk of the lumbosacral plexus can present similarly to an L5 radiculopathy. A plexopathy raises concern of pelvic or retroperitoneal hematoma but can also occur with prolonged labor. Its symptoms can include radicular pain into the foot, frequently in an L5 distribution. Again, a foot drop is a very common finding. Subtle motor involvement on physical exam of S1 weakness, sensory changes on nerve conduction studies, and absence of abnormalities of paraspinal muscles support a diagnosis of plexopathy [58].

Summary

In the hands of an experienced examiner, electrodiagnostic studies, which consist of nerve conduction studies and needle electromyography, are valuable tools for the assessment of patients who have sensory or motor problems in the foot and leg, such as pain, numbness, and weakness. The electrodiagnostic examination is an extension of the physical examination and often provides information that the clinical history and imaging studies do not. A carefully performed electrodiagnostic examination can help to differentiate lumbosacral radiculopathy, plexopathy, focal neuropathy, mononeuropathy, and polyneuropathy, among other conditions. These studies have timing limitations, and do not assess etiology and mechanism, which, if not considered when interpreting the results, can lead to erroneous conclusions. To avoid putting the patient at risk of undergoing an unnecessary procedure or treatment, results should be interpreted cautiously.

References

[1] Kiers L, Clouston P, Zuniga G, et al. Quantitative studies of F responses in Guillian-Barre syndrome and chronic inflammatory demyelinating polyneuropathy. Electroencephalogr Clin Neurophysiol 1994;93(4):255–64.

[2] Aminoff MJ. Clinical electromyography. In: Aminoff MJ, editor. Electrodiagnosis in clinical neurology. 4th edition. New York: Churchill Livingstone; 1999. p. 225–6.

[3] Preston DC, Shapiro BE. Needle electromyography: fundamentals, normal, and abnormal patterns. Neurol Clin North Am 2002;20:361–96.

[4] Wilborn AJ, Aminoff MF. The electrodiagnostic examination in patients with radiculopathies [AAEM Minimonograph 32]. Muscle Nerve 1998;21:1612–31.

[5] Levin KH. Electrodiagnostic approach to the patient with suspected radiculopathy. Neurol Clin North Am 2002;20:397–421.

[6] Shapiro BE, Preston DC. Entrapment and compressive neuropathies. Med Clin North Am 2003;87:663–96.

[7] Katirji B. Lumbosacral radiculopathy. In: Electromyography in clinical practice. St. Louis: Mosby; 1998. p. 13–27.

[8] Levin KH. Low back and neck pain. In: Mancall EL, editor. Neck and back pain. Continuum. Philadelphia: Lippincott, Williams, and Wilkins; 2001. p. 7–43.

[9] Deveraux M. Neck and low back pain. Med Clin N Am 2003;87:643–62.

[10] Linden D, Berlit P. Comparison of late responses, EMG studies, and motor evoked potentials in acute lumbosacral radiculopathies. Muscle Nerve 1995;18:1205–7.

[11] Jensen MC, Brant-Zawadzki MN, Obuchowski N, et al. Magnetic resonance imaging of the lumbar spine in people without back pain. N Engl J Med 1994;331:69–73.

[12] Date ES, Mar EY, Bugola MR, et al. The prevalence of lumbar paraspinal spontaneous activity in asymptomatic subjects. Muscle Nerve 1996;19:350–4.

[13] Dyck PJ, Sinnreich M. Diabetic neuropathies. In: Miller AE, editor. Peripheral neuropathy. Continum. Philadelphia: Lippincott, Williams, and Wilkins; 2003. p. 19–31.

[14] Nobile-Orazio E, Terenghi F. Other dysimmune neuropathies. In: Miller AE, editor. Peripheral neuropathy. Continuum. Philadelphia: Lippincott, Williams, and Wilkins; 2003. p. 56–86.

[15] Wein TH, Albers JW. Electrodiagnostic approach to the patient with suspected peripheral polyneuropathy. Neurol Clin N Am 2002;20:503–26.

[16] Vaillancourt PD, Langevin HM. Painful peripheral neuropathies. Med Clin N Am 1999;83: 627–42.

[17] Wolfe GI, Baker NS, Amato AA, et al. Chronic cryptogenic sensory polyneuropathy. Arch Neurol 1999;56:540–7.

[18] Pastore C, Izura V, Geijo-Barrientos E, et al. A comparison of electrophysiological tests for the early diagnosis of diabetic neuropathy. Muscle Nerve 1999;22:1667–73.

[19] Andersen H, Stalberg E, Falck B. F-wave latency, the most sensitive nerve conduction parameter in patients with diabetes mellitus. Muscle Nerve 1997;20:1296–302.

[20] Killian JM, Foreman PJ. Clinical utility of dorsal sural nerve conduction studies. Muscle Nerve 2001;24:817–20.

[21] Kushnir M, Klein C, Kimiagar Y, et al. Medial dorsal superficial peroneal nerve studies in patients with polyneuropathy and normal sural responses. Muscle Nerve 2004;31:386–9.

[22] Belen J. Orthodromic sensory nerve conduction of the medial and lateral plantar nerves. Am J Phys Med 1985;64:17–23.

[23] DeLisa JA, Saeed MA. The tarsal tunnel syndrome. Muscle Nerve 1983;6:664–70.

[24] Felsenthal G, Butler D, Shear M. Across tarsal tunnel motor nerve conduction technique. Arch Phys Med Rehabil 1992;73:64–9.

[25] Fu R, DeLisa JA, Kraft GH. Motor nerve latencies through the tarsal tunnel in normal adult subjects: standard determinations corrected for temperature and distance. Arch Phys Med Rehabil 1980;61:243–8.

[26] Guiloff RJ, Sherrat RM. Sensory conduction in medial plantar nerve. J Neurol Neurosurg Psychiatry 1977;40:1168–81.

[27] Irani KD, Grabois M, Harvey SC. Standardized technique for diagnosis of tarsal tunnel syndrome. Am J Phys Med 1982;61:26–31.

[28] Johnson EW, Ortiz PR. Electrodiagnosis of tarsal tunnel syndrome. Arch Phys Med Rehabil 1966;47:776–80.

[29] Mondelli M, Giannini F, Reale F. Clinical and electrophysiological findings and follow-up in tarsal tunnel syndrome. Electroencephalogr Clin Neurophysiol 1998;109:418–25.

[30] Oh SJ, Sarala PK, Kuba T, et al. Tarsal tunnel syndrome: electrophysiological study. Ann Neurol 1979;5:327–30.

[31] Ponsford SN. Sensory conduction in medial and lateral plantar nerves. J Neurol Neurosurg Psychiatry 1988;51:188–91.

[32] Saeed MA, Gatens PF. Compound nerve action potentials of the medial and lateral plantar nerves through the tarsal tunnel. Arch Phys Med Rehabil 1982;63:304–7.

[33] Iyer KS, Kaplan E, Goodgold J. Sensory nerve action potentials of the medial and lateral plantar nerve. Arch Phys Med Rehabil 1984;65:529–30.
[34] Park TA, Del Toro DR. The medial calcaneal nerve: anatomy and nerve conduction technique. Muscle Nerve 1995;18:32–8.
[35] Melvin JL, Schuchmann JA, Lanese RR. Diagnostic specificity of motor and sensory nerve conduction variables in the carpal tunnel syndrome. Arch Phys Med Rehabil 1973;54:69–74.
[36] Gatens PF, Saeed MA. Electromyographic findings in the intrinsic muscles of normal feet. Arch Phys Med Rehabil 1982;63:317–8.
[37] Falck B, Alaranta H. Fibrillation potentials, positive sharp waves and fasciculation in the intrinsic muscles of the foot in healthy subjects. J Neurol Neurosurg Psychiatry 1983;46:681–3.
[38] Boon AJ, Harper CM. Needle EMG of abductor hallucis and peroneus tertius in normal subjects. Muscle Nerve 2003;27:752–6.
[39] Adelman KA, Wilson G, Wolf JA. Anterior tarsal tunnel syndrome. J Foot Surg 1988;27:299–302.
[40] Andresen BL, Wertsch JJ, Stewart WA. Anterior tarsal tunnel syndrome. Arch Phys Med Rehabil 1992;73:1112–7.
[41] Borges L, Hallet M, Selkoe D, et al. The anterior tarsal tunnel syndrome. Report of two cases. J Neurosurg 1981;54:89–92.
[42] Krause KH, Witt T, Ross A. The anterior tarsal tunnel syndrome. J Neurol 1977;217:67–74.
[43] Zongzhao L, Jiansheng Z, Li Z. Anterior tarsal tunnel syndrome. J Bone Joint Surg 1991;73B:470–3.
[44] Lambert EH. The accessory deep peroneal nerve. Neurology 1969;19:1169–76.
[45] Lee HJ, Bach JR, DeLisa JA. Deep peroneal sensory nerve: standardization in nerve conduction study. Am J Phys Med Rehabil 1990;69:202–4.
[46] Posas HN, Rivner MH. Nerve conduction studies of the medial branch of the deep peroneal nerve. Muscle Nerve 1990;13:862.
[47] Posas HN, Rivner MH. Deep peroneal sensory neuropathy. Muscle Nerve 1992;15:745–6.
[48] Ponsford S. Medial (cutaneous) branch of deep common peroneal nerve: recording technique and a case report. Electroencephalogr Clin Neurophysiol 1994;93:159–60.
[49] Wiechers D, Guyton JD. Electromyographic findings in the extensor digitorum brevis in a normal population. Arch Phys Med Rehabil 1976;57:84–5.
[50] Rosselle N, Stevens A. Unexpected incidence of neurogenic atrophy of the extensor digitorum brevis muscle in young normal adults. In: Desmedt JE, editor. New developments in electromyography and clinical neurophysiology, vol. 1. Basel (Switzerland): Karger; 1973. p. 69–70.
[51] Izzo KL, Sridhara CR, Rosenholtz H, et al. Sensory conduction studies of the branches of the superficial peroneal nerve. Arch Phys Med Rehabil 1981;62:24–7.
[52] Jabre JF. The superficial peroneal sensory nerve revisited. Arch Neurol 1981;38:666–7.
[53] Levin KH, Stevens JC, Daube JR. Superficial peroneal nerve conduction studies for electromyographic diagnosis. Muscle Nerve 1986;9:322–6.
[54] Oh SJ, Demirci M, Dajani B, et al. Distal sensory nerve conduction of the superficial peroneal nerve: new method and its clinical application. Muscle Nerve 2001;24:689–94.
[55] Sridhara CR, Izzo KL. Terminal sensory branches of the superficial peroneal nerve: an entrapment syndrome. Arch Phys Med Rehabil 1985;66:789–91.
[56] DiBenedetto M. Sensory nerve conduction in lower extremities. Arch Phys Med Rehabil 1970;51:253–8 285.
[57] Katirji B. Sciatic neuropathy. In: Electromyography in clinical practice. St. Louis: Mosby; 1998. p. 29–38.
[58] Katirji B. Lumbosacral plexopathy. In: Electromyography in clinical practice. St. Louis: Mosby; 1998. p. 47–62.

ELSEVIER
SAUNDERS

Clin Podiatr Med Surg
23 (2006) 545–557

CLINICS IN
PODIATRIC
MEDICINE AND
SURGERY

Quantitative Sensory Testing

David Soomekh, DPM[a,b]

[a]The Foot and Ankle Institute of Santa Monica, Santa Monica, CA, USA
[b]Clinical Instructor, UCLA Medical Center, Santa Monica, CA, USA

The diagnosis and treatment of peripheral neuropathy from any cause has come to the forefront of the research community in the past few years. Both past and new diagnostic and treatment options have been and are being studied to better understand and properly treat this debilitating and sometimes devastating disease. One such advancement is the clinical use of quantitative sensory testing. To identify etiology, quality, pattern, and degree of the neuropathy early, the testing instrument would need to identify changes throughout the course of the disease, have a normative database, and show a clear distinction between the absence or presence of disease [1]. The pressure specified sensory device (PSSD; Sensory Management Services, LLC, Baltimore, MD) was developed in 1992 to painlessly investigate the cutaneous pressure thresholds quantitatively and accurately.

Anatomy and nerve injury

The peripheral nerve is composed of motor, sensory, and sympathetic nerve fibers. The cell body of the fibers of the motor nerve resides in the anterior horn and of the spinal cord and terminates at the neuromuscular junction in the muscle. The cell body of the presynaptic sympathetic nerve fibers resides within the anterior horn as well. The sensory nerve cell body lies in the dorsal root ganglia and then terminates in the skin as free nerve endings or in specialized group receptors [2].

Nerve injury can be described as and classified into six different types (Figs. 1–4). Seddon [3] in 1943 described the first three types: neuropraxia, axonotmesis, and neurotmesis. In 1951 Sunderland [4] went on to add two more classifications that precede neurotmesis. In 1988 Dellon [5] described one more classification of injury that combines nerve injury of various

---

The Foot and Ankle Institute of Santa Monica, Santa Monica, CA.
E-mail address: david@footankleinstitute.com

doi:10.1016/j.cpm.2006.05.005

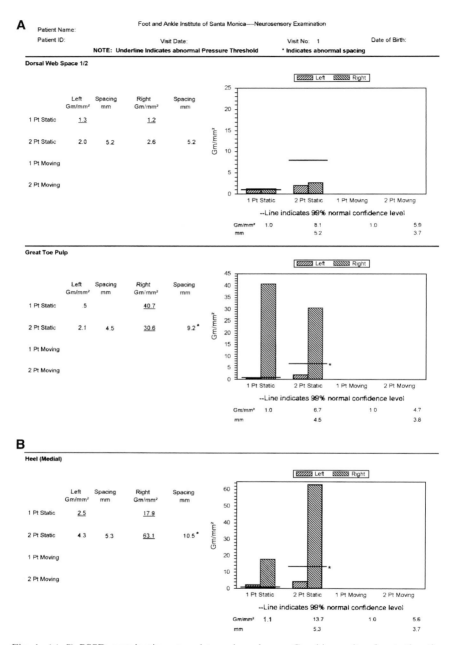

Fig. 1. (*A–B*) PSSD examination—tarsal tunnel syndrome. Graphic results after testing the dorsal web space, the great toe pulp and the medial heel for a patient presenting with heel and arch pain on the right foot. There is an increased amount of pressure needed for a response on the right side for both one-point and two-point testing at the great toe and the medial heel. There is also an increase in the widening of the two points for both locations from a normal of 4.5 mm to 9.2 mm at the great toe, and from a normal of 5.3 mm to 10.5 mm at the medial heel. This shows a relatively significant right-sided tarsal tunnel syndrome with axonal loss.

degrees from fascicle to fascicle. The classification can then be thought of as six degrees of nerve injury (Table 1).

Neuropraxia or first-degree injury involves a block in the conduction at a certain point along the course of the nerve. There are no changes to the nerve's morphology histopathologically. The nerve will lose its ability to conduct the impulse just at the damaged nerve fiber. Clinically the nerve may look normal. The recovery from this injury is complete over days to weeks. Once the nerve restores its block of conduction, the recovery will be immediate. This is in part because there is no myelin disruption nor is there axonal damage. Without axonal damage, there is no nerve regeneration that needs to take place. Since there is no axonal damage there will be no Tinel's sign. Any type of early nerve entrapment or compression will lead to this first-degree injury [5].

Axonotmesis or second-degree injury involves damage to the axon. There is enough destruction that leads to distal segment Wallerian degeneration. The proximal segment will undergo regeneration of the axon by sprouting. In this case then, actual nerve regeneration will take place. For this reason there will be a Tinel's sign noted at the site of injury and then move distally as it heals. There will be full recovery from this type of injury to the nerve, as the endoneurium and perineurium are spared. The differentiation between this axonotmesis and first degree is the time in which full recovery is achieved. A diagnosis of neuropraxia is made at 3 months and earlier while axonotmesis is over this time point [5].

Third-degree injury is then an axonotmesis with an incomplete recovery. The key to this type of injury is the disruption of the endoneurium. As the nerve fibers regenerate they must then pass through scar tissue. The ends of many of the fibers are then unable to make contact with their receptors or end organs as they become trapped within the scar tissue. The disruption of the Schwann cells leads to some fibers healing to the improper distal fiber. This event can then cause some sensory fibers to make contact with motor fibers if the injury is proximal within the extremity. If the injury is distal in the extremity, this mismatch is less likely and the injury will be all sensory or all motor, leading to a better incomplete recovery than the aforementioned [5].

Fourth-degree injury is described by those nerves that remain intact after the injury, yet have no function or restoration. The nerve is held together solely within the scar tissue. The distal innervations are then affected by incomplete function. There will be a Tinel's sign seen at the level of injury only. To have any recovery take place, surgical repair is needed [5].

Fifth-degree injury is identified by complete transaction of the peripheral nerve [5]. Surgical management of these injuries can result in some recovery.

Sixth-degree injury, or what Dellon calls neuroma incontinuity, is described as an injury to the nerve that presents injury to some fascicles with mixed degrees of injury and normal function through other fascicles within the same nerve fiber. This will then lead to mixed recovery in the innervated area and a poor recovery.

Nerve compression

The most common pathologic process in the lower extremity involving nerve injury lies with nerve compression. This can also be described as

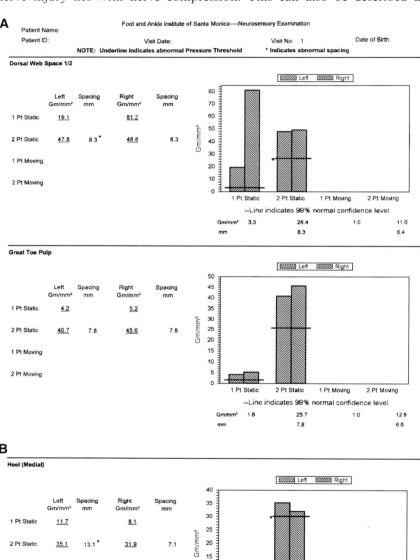

entrapment neuropathy. It then becomes important to have a good under-standing of the pathology of the nerve under compression and more specif-ically, chronic compression. The nerve fibers will go through many of the degrees of injury covered above. The outer fibers of the fascicles are dam-aged first, while the central fibers remain intact and undamaged early in the compression. As the entrapment continues, Wallerian degeneration be-gins to the large myelinated fibers [5]. The amount of injury is then directly related to the degree and duration of the compression.

Nerve compression can be caused by edema surrounding the nerve exter-nally, edema within the nerve, or external compression from other anatomical structures in the area. There is variability in the severity of injury depending on acute or chronic compression of the nerve. The A-beta fibers (large diam-eter) are the most susceptible to compression and ischemia. One will first note a loss of circumferential A-beta fibers. Mechanical and ischemic factors can also impair the function of the nerve. Microcirculation and axoplasmic trans-port are then inhibited, intraneural scar formation and edema and eventually fiber degeneration and death will occur. Static touch on the skin is translated by Merkle cells with slow-adapting A-beta nerve fibers. Moving touch is translated by Miessner corpuscles, which have quickly adapting A-beta nerve fibers. Diminished oxygen slows axonal transport leading to disruption to the A-beta fibers and loss of light touch. With compression, there is a drop out circumferentially of the large diameter A-beta fibers.

For the Merkle cell there are three to eight receptors to an A-beta fiber. For the Miessner cell there are two to eight A-beta fibers to one receptor. This means that when there is damage to the nerve, the first sensation to be lost is the static two-point discrimination, and the first to return with nerve regeneration is one point moving touch. With this knowledge, one can then understand that static measurement should be performed to deter-mine the extent of damage while to evaluate the rate of healing, interpreta-tion of moving touch tests should be made.

Diagnosis

Measuring the loss of motor function is well documented and relatively easy to assess and diagnose weakness with manual muscle examination.

Fig. 2. (A–B) PSSD examination—medial calcaneal nerve entrapment. Graphic results after test-ing the dorsal web space, the great toe pulp, and the medial heel for a patient presenting with left heel pain mimicking plantar fascitis. The horizontal line through the bars indicates the normal value. The asterisk next to the bar indicates a widening of the distance between the two points dur-ing two-point testing. In this patient the medial left heel shows a widening of the two points from a normal of 7.1 mm to 13.1 mm. This is an indication of axonal damage. There is also an increase in the pressure needed to get a response from the patient in both the one point and the two point compared with the contralateral side. Although the dorsal web space value for the left foot is also widened about 1 mm, the patient had no symptoms in this area. The great toe results are relatively normal. This shows a relatively significant medial calcaneal nerve entrapment.

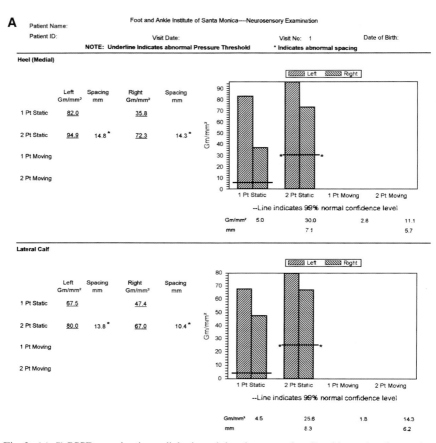

Fig. 3. (*A–B*) PSSD examination—diabetic peripheral neuropathy. Graphic results after testing the dorsal web space, the great toe pulp, the medial heel, and the lateral calf for a patient presenting with diabetic neuropathy symptoms bilaterally. All values are shown to be increased bilaterally both with one-point and two-point discrimination worse on the left than the right. There is also a significant widening of the distance between the two points in all areas bilateral extending up to the lateral calf. This shows a very significant bilateral peripheral neuropathy worse on the left than the right with significant axonal loss.

Sensory loss is more difficult to evaluate. In the early stages of sensory loss owing to compression there will be an increased hypersensitivity response to a stimulus. As the compression progresses, the intensity of the stimulus needs to increase to elicit a response. This can be tested with vibratory testing and or cutaneous pressure threshold testing. Sensory loss can be equivocated to motor atrophy and wasting as irregular two-point discrimination.

Tinel's sign is also a helpful clinical examination. As mentioned earlier, the appearance of a Tinel's sign will only be in the event of nerve degeneration and so will be present during the course of regeneration with a nerve compression. So, with minimal compression when there is no degeneration,

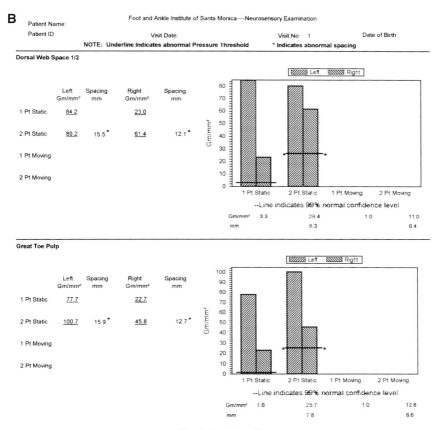

Fig. 3 (*continued*)

the sign will be negative. As the entrapment and damage increases, the sign will become positive. Severe compression or prolonged damage without resultant regeneration will then show a negative Tinel's sign [5].

Electrodiagnostic testing is very valuable in the diagnosis and determination of degree of damage to peripheral nerves if used in the proper situations and with an understanding of its limitations. The primary use of these tests should be reserved for when the clinician has been unable to make a proper diagnosis through the patient's clinical manifestations and they have ruled out systemic causes of peripheral neuropathy such as diabetes or alcoholism. These studies are helpful in making a determination between peripheral neuropathy and myopathy.

The problem arises with electrodiagnostic studies with the high incidence of those patients with obvious clinical symptoms when the examination is a "normal" study [11]. In one study it was found that nerve conduction velocity (NCV) tests had a sensitivity of 80% and a specificity of 77% while

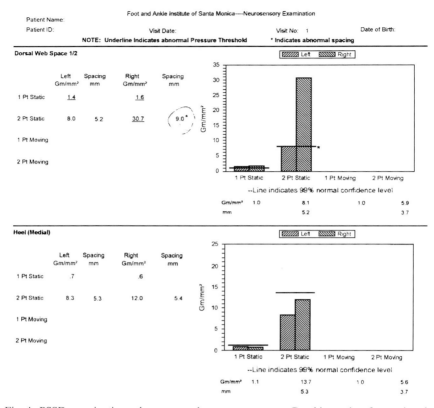

Fig. 4. PSSD examination—deep peroneal nerve entrapment. Graphic results after testing the
dorsal web space and the medial heel for a patient presenting with pain and numbness within
the first innerspace of the right foot. The horizontal line through the bars indicates the normal
value. The asterisk next to the bar indicates a widening of the distance between the two points
during two-point testing. All the results are normal except for the right dorsal innerspace on
two-point discrimination with a widening of the two points from a normal of 5.2 mm to 9.0
mm. There is also an increased amount of pressure applied before the patient responds. This
shows a relatively significant deep peroneal nerve entrapment.

the PSSD had a sensitivity of 91% and a specificity of 82% for carpal tunnel
syndrome [5]. Although this difference was not shown to be significant, the
pain experienced by the patients was far less with the PSSD. Another study
concluded that the PSSD has a high sensitivity but a low specificity when
compared with electrodiagnostic testing in the diagnosis of a peripheral nerve
entrapment [6]. False negative NCV test results for tarsal tunnel syndrome
are upwards of 50% and 30% for carpal tunnel syndrome [7]. With nerve
conduction studies it is not possible clearly identify the specific branches
that are affected from the posterior tibial nerve in tarsal tunnel syndrome.
Mackinnon and Dellon [8] relate that a normal study cannot be an absolute
contraindication to surgical decompression nor can an abnormal study be

Table 1
Classification of nerve injuries

Degree of injury	Histopathologic changes					Tinel Sign	
	Myelin	Axon	Endoneurium	Perineurium	Epineurium	Present	Progresses distally
I Neuropraxia	+/−					−	−
II Axonotmesis	+	+				+	+
III	+	+	+			+	+
IV	+	+	+	+		+	−
V Neurotmesis	+	+	+	+	+	+	−
VI	Various fibers & fascicles demonstrate various pathologic changes					+	+/−

Courtesy of A. Lee Dellon, MD, Baltimore, Maryland.

a clear indication that surgery is needed. Many studies have demonstrated that with the event of chronic nerve compression there can be mixed damage to the different fascicles within the nerve. This can then lead to motor loss without sensory loss or sensory loss without motor loss resulting in many false negatives with the testing [5]. The electrodes of the device will usually measure the fastest conducting fibers and will not reveal the one or two damaged fascicles in the area again resulting in a false negative study. Even the patient's body temperature and the ambient temperature will affect the result of the examination. Most importantly, the studies are less sensitive to early damage when compared with pressure threshold studies.

The traditional 5.07 Semmes Weinstein monofilament test provides only an estimated range of the force applied, not a true measurement. The filament bends at a pressure of 95 g/mm^2. It has been shown that diabetic patients are susceptible to skin breakdown at a level of 30 g/mm^2 [9–11]. Studies have shown that there is a great deal of variation in the force able to bend the filament. This can be because of errors in the application of the unit, temperature changes, and the differing makeup and assembly of the filament on the handle. There is also a great deal of misinterpretation of the results.

Quantitative sensory testing

Quantitative sensory testing is a term that is used to define the diagnostic tools used to measure temperature perception thresholds (a function of small myelinated nerve fibers) and for perception of pressure and vibratory thresholds (a function of the large myelinated nerve fibers) [7]. With nerve compression the small myelinated fibers and their function are lost after the function of the large myelinated fibers. Therefore it was important to develop a test that can examine the degree of injury based on touch or pressure threshold as it will be lost first and regained in recovery last. Dellon and his group developed such a technique.

The PSSD can measure the cutaneous pressure thresholds in a manner that is inexpensive and painless. It can measure the thresholds for perception of one-point static touch and one point moving across the skin. It can also measure the perception of static two-point discrimination and moving two-point discrimination and the pressure needed to perceive the two-point discrimination.

Two-point discrimination testing evaluates the slowly adapting fibers' receptor system [1]. This system is programmed by intensity or by increasing spatial recruitment of the neighboring fibers. There is then the need to examine the patient's ability to distinguish that there are two points of touch at a certain distance apart while also measuring the amount of pressure needed to be applied before the discrimination at the specified distance can be made. The patient's ability to distinguish between one and two points of pressure is related to the number of axons innervating the cutaneous area [1]. Distinguishing two points of pressure then becomes important in evaluating the extent of axonal damage. Furthermore, this perception is the first to become abnormal with a nerve compression.

With one-point sensory testing, one is testing for the level of sensory function. Pressure thresholds above normal indicate abnormal functioning of touch receptors and the nerve fibers innervating those receptors. With two-point sensory testing, one is measuring the level of innervation density. Two-point discrimination wider than normal indicates the loss of receptors and degeneration of nerve fibers. As the patient's ability to distinguish two points of pressure decreases when the two points are brought closer together, there is then more severity of axonal damage and death to the nerve and more aggressive treatment would be indicated. The loss of sensibility is to the sensory nerve what weakness is to muscle. The loss of innervation density is to sensory nerve what atrophy is to muscle.

The PSSD works by measuring the pressure applied to a cutaneous area. There is a force transducer within the handheld device behind each of the two prongs. Each transducer can measure the perception of the pressure against it in a range from 0.1 g/mm^2 to 100 g/mm^2. As the force is applied to the device, the computer attached to the hand piece will record the increase in pressure live graphically. The examiner is then able to inspect the rate at which he or she is increasing the pressure. The patient will have a button in his or her hand that when pressed stops the computer from measuring the continuing increase in pressure and records the end point force. The examiner will choose the site, right or left, and the type of exam wanted. The same test site for the same test type will be tested five times. The computer then throws out the highest and the lowest force values and calculates a mean of the remaining three values.

Normal values of cutaneous pressures for various areas of the extremities stratified by age for both one-point and two-point discrimination with the separation distances between the prongs have been evaluated and are stored in the software. When evaluating the results of the examination, they can be compared both to "normal" and to the contralateral extremity. There will be a line of the graph that will show the normal pressure value and a bar that shows the patient's value for that specific examination. The "y" axis of the graph will show an increase in pressure as it rises and the "x" axis shows the type of exam taken. All the values for the right extremity are indicated in red and the left extremity are in blue. When testing for two-point discrimination, if there is a need to increase the distance between the prongs an asterisk will be placed by the bar. All the numeric values will also be shown on the graph.

A patient with normal cutaneous thresholds will need less pressure from the device while an abnormal threshold would require more pressure from the device, and a higher value on the graph. A patient with normal one-point discrimination and high two-point discrimination with normal distance between the prongs can be said to have mild pathology to the nerve. Moderate damage would be shown with high levels for both the one- and two-point discrimination. When distance between the prongs increases before the patient can distinguish two-point discrimination the nerve is becoming severely damaged and there is said to be significant axonal damage. The farther apart the prongs are from normal, the more significant the disease.

The test sites chosen are based on the pathology that is being ruled out (Table 2). The one-point static and two-point static testing should be used to make a diagnosis and determine if the course of treatment should be conservative or surgical decompression. The device can be used to evaluate systemic causes of peripheral neuropathy like diabetic and alcoholic peripheral neuropathy, tarsal tunnel syndrome, carpal tunnel syndrome, interdigital neuroma or entrapment, common peroneal nerve entrapment, cubital tunnel syndrome, deep peroneal nerve entrapment and others. The testing can be used for sensibility over time as well. For example, if over two testing periods there is an increase in the pressure threshold yet no change in the two-point discrimination distance, then there is a worsening of the nerve's function. If between testing times the pressure threshold for two-point discrimination remains the same and the two-point discrimination distance increases, then there is a loss of nerve fibers and a worsening of nerve function [2].

The PSSD can also be used to evaluate the regeneration of the nerve after microsurgery or nerve decompression over time. This would be the time to use the one-point moving and two-point moving tests. As the physiology of nerve regeneration and repair has shown us, the first parameter to be restored is the cutaneous pressure threshold for one-point moving and then one-point static and then two-point moving and then two-point static [7].

Table 2
Testing areas as related to potential diagnosis

	Great toe pulp	Medial heel	Dorsal 1st innerspace	Lateral calf
Diabetic neuropathy	X	X	X	X
Tarsal tunnel syndrome	X	X	X	
Neuroma			X	
Common peroneal	X	X		X

If the subject has a recovery pattern that is different form this, for example the one-point moving and one-point static recover but the two-point moving does not, it can be assumed that there is a block in the progression of the recovery. The examination is also very useful during a limb lengthening. As the limb is lengthened, the degree of distraction each day will be limited by the amount of nerve growth and vessel elongation. To ensure the degree of distraction is correct and not too fast, the PSSD test can be performed throughout the course of the lengthening .

The following is an example of the procedure followed for a routine examination to test for tarsal tunnel syndrome in the right lower extremity using the PSSD. The patient should be made very familiar with the examination and given proper instructions. The author will tell the patient that he will conduct the one-point test first and that at the instant the patient feels any sort of touch to the given area, the button should be pressed. The patient is told not to expect a certain type of a feeling, nor should he or she expect the sensation to feel like what the prongs look like they should feel. They may feel as though the sensation is one of very hard pressure, light touch, a feather, water, cloth, or even the examiner's finger. The patient is told that the computer will make an audible tone when the button is pressed and the force value is recorded. This tells the patient that the author has taken the pressure device off the area and will then repeat the examination four more times. The patient is then told that at the same site, after the one-point test is finished, the two-point test will be given. The patient is told that he or she should not press the button this time at the instant a sensation is felt, yet to wait until able to distinguish that there are two points of touch to the area, and that this will take more time and pressure to feel than did the one-point test. The patient is reminded that simply feeling a lot of pressure does not mean that he or she feels two points of sensation. The patient is told that if he or she cannot distinguish the two points not to press the button, and that the examiner will increase the distance between the points and attempt the examination again repeating this until he or she is able to feel the second point. The author will make the patient familiar with the sensation of two points by showing what it feels like on the patient's index finger. The patient will sit in the examination chair with his or her eyes closed or the testing area hidden from view. The great toe pulp is tested first with both one-point testing and then two-point discrimination, followed by the medial heel and the dorsal first innerspace. The unaffected side should be tested first to give the patient the chance to "learn" the test. There are those patients who believe they are feeling two points when they are only really feeling one. The examiner can reduce for this margin of error during the two-point test by only placing one prong on the test area every so often. The patient may then press the button, and because the software will not register a value or sound a tone when two-point testing is chosen and only one prong is used, the patient will likely advise you that the button does not seem to be working. This is how you can evaluate the patient's ability to understand the instructions.

The author has found that there is a large learning curve in the patient population for understanding the examination. This is why it is important to take the time to explain the exam thoroughly and to repeat the instructions throughout the examinations many times. The software will also allow for deleting trials if the examiner feels a trial may be poor.

Summary

The PSSD is a very useful tool in ruling out compression syndromes and peripheral neuropathy. It is also a powerful tool for identifying and quantifying the degree of nerve recovery. It has become reproducible and consistent in the author's use. When there is no axonal loss, an attempt at conservative care with physical therapy is warranted. In the presence of axonal damage, surgical exploration and decompression may be warranted. The author will use the device to determine the need for conservative care versus surgical decompression with caution. Clinical correlation with imaging and other diagnostic tools should be used in conjunction with PSSD results. The use of the PSSD should not deter the clinician from acquiring additional electrodiagnostic studies as well.

References

[1] Barber MA, Conolley J, Spaulding CM, et al. Evaluation of pressure threshold prior to foot ulceration. JAPMA 2001;91(10):508–14.

[2] Aszmann OC, Dellon AL. Relationship between cutaneous pressure threshold and two-point discrimination. J Reconstr Microsurg 1998;14(6):417–21.

[3] Seddon HJ. Three types of nerve injury. Brain 1943;66:237.

[4] Sunderland S. A classification of peripheral nerve injuries producing loss of function. Brain 1951;74:491.

[5] Weber RA, Schuchmann JA, Albers JH, et al. A prospective blinded evaluation of nerve conduction velocity versus pressure-specified sensory testing in carpal tunnel syndrome. Ann Plast Surg 2000;45(3):252–7.

[6] Tassler PL, Dellon AL. Pressure perception in the normal lower extremity and in tarsal tunnel syndrome. Muscle Nerve 1996;19:285–9.

[7] Dellon AL. Management of peripheral nerve problems in the upper and lower extremity using quantitative sensory testing. Hand Clin 1999;15(4):697–715.

[8] Mackinnon SE, Dellon AL. Surgery of the peripheral nerve. New York: Thieme Medical Publishers Inc; 1988;108.

[9] Dellon ES, Crone S, Mouery R, et al. Comparison of the Semmes Weinstein monofilaments with the pressure-specifying sensory device. Restor Neurol Neurosci 1993;5:323–6.

[10] Dellon ES, Mourry R, Dellon AL. Human pressure perception values for constant and move one and two-point discrimination. Plast Reconstr Surg 1992;90:112–7.

[11] Tassler PL, Dellon AL. Correlation of measuements of pressure perception using the pressure-specifying sensory device with electrodiagnositic testing. JOEM 1995;37:862–6.

ELSEVIER
SAUNDERS

Clin Podiatr Med Surg
23 (2006) 559–567

CLINICS IN
PODIATRIC
MEDICINE AND
SURGERY

Prognostic Ability of a Good Outcome to Carpal Tunnel Release for Decompression Surgery in the Lower Extremity

Christopher T. Maloney, Jr, MD*, A. Lee Dellon, MD,
Christopher Heller, Jr, BS, Joshua R. Olson, BS

*The Institute for Plastic Surgery and Peripheral Nerve Surgery,
3170 N. Swan Road, Tucson, Arizona 85712, USA*

Many patients who have neuropathy present with pain and numbness in a glove and stocking distribution. For years, patients who were treated successfully with carpal tunnel release were told there was nothing that could be done about their lower extremity symptoms. Now that lower extremity nerve decompression has been accepted as an option to treat appropriate patients, the authors looked for correlations between a successful outcome with carpal tunnel syndrome and its predictive value of success for lower extremity nerve decompression. The hypothesis tested is that a good outcome from carpal tunnel decompression will correlate with, or be a predictor of, a good result from lower extremity peripheral nerve decompression.

Within diabetes mellitus, there are many forms of neuropathy. The distal, large fiber, symmetrical polyneuropathy is the most common form [1,2]. The natural history of this form of diabetic neuropathy is well described, and, in the western world, has remained unchanged for more than half a century and in studies that include more than 30,000 people who have diabetes [3–11]. For example, in the study of 4400 diabetes patients reported by Pirart in 1944, neuropathy was present in 12% at the time of diagnosis, and increased to 50% by the time diabetes had been present for 25 years [12]. Loss of sensibility leads to infection, ulceration, and amputation, which is independent from the amputations because of large vessel disease [13].

* Corresponding author.
E-mail address: chrismaloney2@yahoo.com (C.T. Maloney, Jr).

0891-8422/06/$ - see front matter © 2006 Elsevier Inc. All rights reserved.
doi:10.1016/j.cpm.2006.04.008

The incidence of ulceration is 2.5% per year and occurs in one of six diabetes patients in their lifetime [14–17]. Even the Diabetic Control and Complication Trail, for which the goal was euglycemia, did not prevent the occurrence of diabetic neuropathy, although the incidence was reduced [18]. The loss of sensibility also results in balance problems which can lead to falls and hip and wrist fractures [17–20]. Individuals who have a painful component to their neuropathy require neuropathic pain medication, often to the extent that there are such cognitive changes the patient becomes disabled related to the pain component of the neuropathy alone [21–28]. Non-healing ulcers precede 80%–85% of amputations in patients who have neuropathy [29,30]. Despite various strategies to decrease the number of amputations in the United States (eg, better glucose control, monitoring screening exams for impaired sensibility), the number of amputations has continued to increase from 54,000 in 1990 [31], to 92,000 in 1999 [32]. The average cost of ulceration was $27,500 in 1997 and the cost of an amputation ranges from $22,702 for a toe, to $51,281 for a leg. The annual cost for diabetic neuropathy and its complications in the United States is between $4.6 and $13.7 billion [33,34]. It is estimated that up to 27% of the direct medical costs of diabetes mellitus are related to diabetic neuropathy [34]. There are estimated to be 16 million individuals who have diabetes in the United States and this number is expected to double by 2030 [35]. The number is increasing in epidemic proportions because the overweight population is developing insulin resistance [36–38]. According to the Centers for Disease Control and Prevention, "During 2000–2002, an estimated 11.7% of U.S. adults with diabetes had a history of foot ulcer [39]." Although the natural history of diabetic neuropathy is well documented, diabetic neuropathy is progressive and irreversible [40]. There are two metabolic changes in the peripheral nerves of an individual who has diabetes that render the nerve susceptible to chronic compression. The most critical is the increased water content within the nerve which results when glucose is metabolized into sorbitol [41]. This increased water content causes the nerve to increase in volume. The second metabolic change is a decrease in the slow anterograde component of axoplasmic flow [42]. This component of axoplasmic flows transports the lipoproteins necessary to maintain and rebuild the nerve. The peripheral nerve, as it crosses a known area of anatomic narrowing (eg, the carpal tunnel at the wrist, the cubital tunnel at the elbow, the fibular tunnel at the outside of the knee, the tarsal tunnel at the ankle), passes through a region of increased external pressure. In individuals who have diabetes, the peripheral nerve has an increased volume because of its water content, and therefore, there is increased pressure on the nerve in each of these anatomic regions.

   This increased external pressure creates an increased intraneural pressure, which decreases blood flow and results in a relative ischemic condition for the peripheral nerve [43]. The neurophysiologic consequence of decreased blood flow in a peripheral nerve is the perception of paresthesias, interpreted centrally as numbness and tingling. The chronic pathophysiologic result of this area of increased pressure along a peripheral nerve is demyelination. The peripheral nerve that has decreased axoplasmic flow (ie, as in people who have diabetes), cannot transport sufficient protein structures to rebuild itself. Additionally, advanced glycosylation end products reduce the normal gliding ability of the peripheral nerve. The non-enzymatic binding of glucose to the collagen within the nerve and in the epineurium is the basis for this decreased elasticity. The combination of this decreased elasticity in the peripheral nerve, combined with the nerve's normal physiologic requirement to stretch as it glides across joints, increases the stress and strain of the peripheral nerve within these areas of known anatomic narrowing. This increased tension along the nerve further decreases blood flow within the nerve [44].

The hypothesis that the peripheral nerve in a person with diabetes has an increased susceptibility to compression has been tested in the rat model [45]. Rats were made diabetic by being given streptozotocin. Silicone bands were placed about the sciatic nerve in these rats, and also in a group of non-diabetic, age-matched rats. Electrophysiology was tested in both groups after 6 months of banding; sufficient time to develop electrophysiological and histological changes consistent with chronic nerve compression in this model [46]. The diabetic rat had a statistically significant lower conduction velocity and a statistically significant lower amplitude for the sciatic nerve measured across the region of compression than did the non-diabetic banded rat. The study confirmed that the peripheral nerve has an increased susceptibility to chronic nerve compression in the diabetic rat.

Chemotherapy is also a common cause of peripheral neuropathy. Plastic surgeons encounter clinical problems related to cisplatin and tactual chemotherapy. Most often these problems are related to soft-tissue injury that results from extravasation of the drug during intravenous infusion therapy [47,48]. Cisplatin [49–51] and paclitaxel [52–54], however, each cause a painful chemotherapy-induced neuropathy which results from their binding to tubulin in the axoplasm. This causes a decrease in the slow component of anterograde axoplasmic transport that makes the peripheral nerve susceptible to chronic nerve compression. In a study from 1984, postmortem histological examination demonstrated concentrations of cisplatin in the peripheral nerve at the same level as in the tumor, approximately 3 µg/g, whereas the cisplatin levels in the central nervous system were low, approximately 0.2 µg/g, because cisplatin does not cross through the blood-brain barrier [49]. A similar mechanism in diabetes results in a susceptibility to chronic nerve compression [55,56] that can be reversed by decompression of the peripheral nerve [57]. Clinical success with this approach has resulted in restoration of sensation and relief of pain in 80% of patients, including both upper and lower extremity nerve compression sites [58–61]. This subject has been reviewed recently [62]. Similar success in the basic science model of cisplatin neuropathy in the rat [63] provided a basis to apply this approach to patients who have disabling symptoms of chemotherapy-induced neuropathy [64].

As mention earlier, in patients with diabetic neuropathy there is increased incidence of peripheral nerve compression. The most recent report related to this observation [65], which was for median nerve compression in the carpal tunnel, demonstrated a 2% incidence of carpal tunnel syndrome in the population with no diabetes, 14% in the population who had diabetes without neuropathy, and 30% in the population who had diabetes with neuropathy.

The diabetic patient with neuropathy has symptoms that include sensory complaints such as numbness and tingling, pain, loss of sensation, and motor complaints like weakness. The motor complaints extend to the autonomic system as well, and in the extremities, include loss of sudomotor function, so the skin becomes dry and thick. The sensory symptoms occur in a distribution that has been called "stocking and glove"; the symptoms are worse in the lower extremity than the upper extremity. In contrast, the patient who has a single chronic nerve compression will have these same symptoms; however, they will occur only in the distribution of that particular nerve. For example, the patient who has carpal tunnel syndrome, with median nerve compression, will only have the sensory complaints in the palmar aspect of the thumb, index, and middle finger, and will only have weakness in the muscles that control part of the thumb's function [66]. In the upper extremity, chronic compression of the ulnar nerve at the elbow will result in paresthesias in the palmar and dorsal surfaces of the ring and little finger, and weakness of pinch and grip strength. In advanced cases of ulnar nerve compression, there is intrinsic muscle weakness, which creates a claw-like deformity of the hand. Ulnar nerve compression at the elbow can be decompressed surgically [67,68]. If the radial sensory nerve were compressed in the forearm, there would be numbness over the remaining skin surface of the hand, the dorsoradial skin. The radial sensory nerve can be decompressed surgically, too [69]. If a person were to have chronic compression of the median, ulnar and radial nerves, that person would have a glove distribution of numbness, and have symptoms indistinguishable from the patient with symptomatic diabetic neuropathy of the upper extremity.

This same relationship applies to the lower extremity. Compression of the sciatic nerve's common peroneal nerve at the lateral aspect of the knee occurs in the fibular tunnel. The symptoms include paresthesia, or pain from the knee to the top of the foot. The motor component, when complete, results in a drop foot, and complete compression of the motor branch of the radial nerve, at the elbow, results in a drop wrist. More commonly, in the leg, there is weakness of the long toe extensor, so this toe is positioned lower than the other toes, and is weak on manual muscle testing [70]. Compression of the common peroneal nerve in this location requires a neurolysis by division of the fascial coverings above and below the peroneus longus muscle. Over the dorsum of the foot, the deep peroneal nerve can be entrapped between the extensor digitorum brevis and the junction of the first metatarsal and the cunieform bone [71]. This entrapment is corrected by excising the tendon of this small muscle, which has no functional significance in the foot. Entrapment of the deep peroneal nerve is similar to the radial sensory nerve entrapment in the forearm. The analogy of the carpal tunnel syndrome in the foot is the tarsal tunnel syndrome [72,73]. However, it must be realized that the tarsal tunnel is really the analogy of the human forearm, and therefore, to achieve restoration of sensation of all toes and the plantar aspect of the foot, the medial and lateral plantar nerves and the calcaneal nerve must each be released in their own separate tunnels, just distal to the tarsal tunnel. It is severe compression of the lateral plantar nerve that creates the hyperextended toes at the metatarsal phalangeal joints. These appear as "hammer toes" in a person who has diabetes, but are really claw-like toes, caused by intrinsic muscle paralysis in the foot, just like the claw-like hand results from intrinsic muscle paralysis in the hand [74]. Relief of paresthesias and pain in the foot, and often correction of the intrinsic muscle wasting, can be accomplished by decompression of the four medial ankle tunnels [75]. If a person were to have chronic compression of the peroneal and tibial nerves, that person would have a stocking distribution of numbness, and have symptoms indistinguishable from the patient with symptomatic diabetic neuropathy of the lower extremity.

How can a physician identify compression of the peripheral nerve? The most reliable clinical finding of a nerve compression is tenderness of the nerve at the site of anatomic narrowing. This sensitivity of the nerve at the site of chronic compression may be manifested simply by the nerve being tender at that site, but most often is manifested by a distally radiating paresthesia in the distribution of the nerve when the nerve is gently percussed. This is referred to as a positive Tinel sign [76]. In a patient with a neuropathy, where a systemic cause exists for the nerve dysfunction, there should be no localizing sign along the course of the peripheral nerve. However, if the neuropathy causes the nerve to be susceptible to nerve compression, then there can be superimposed compression of the peripheral nerve in addition to the underlying neuropathy. Traditionally, electrodiagnostic testing is used to make the diagnosis of peripheral nerve compression, neuropathy, or nerve root compression. There are many times, however, when the peripheral neuropathy is so advantaged that there is no conduction measurable in the peripheral nerve, or the conduction velocity and amplitude are already so reduced, that identification of a superimposed nerve compression in the patient with neuropathy is just not possible technically. In these situations, the physical examination is critical to make this distinction [62].

A retrospective cohort study was designed from a database of 300 patients who had previous decompression of lower extremity peripheral nerves to restore sensation and relieve pain in their feet. Inclusion criteria for the study were (1) history of carpal tunnel decompression before the date of the lower extremity peripheral nerve surgery, and (2) presence of peripheral neuropathy. Patients who had neuropathy as a result of diabetes mellitus, chemotherapy, or unknown etiology were included. Thirty-five patients were selected for this study. Original consultation notes were reviewed to determine the patient's stated outcome to their carpal tunnel surgery and this answer, dichotomized into either a good/excellent or fair/poor result was compared with their dichotomized result from their lower extremity peripheral nerve surgery. Outcome for the surgery was predicated upon improvement in pain or recovery of sensation, as determined by the patient's office visit interview. Statistical analysis was done for sensitivity, specificity, and positive predictive value. Thirty-four of the 35 patients had a good/excellent response to the carpal tunnel release. Their sensation increased and any pain or numbness they previously had was gone. Thirty of the 34 patients who had a good response to carpal tunnel release had a good/excellent response to lower extremity peripheral nerve decompression. These patients reported increased sensation and their pain disappeared completely or decreased significantly. Analysis of this study data resulted in 97% sensitivity, 0% specificity, and 88% positive predictive value. The most important implication of this result is that in the patient who has peripheral neuropathy, 88% who have a good outcome from carpal tunnel decompression can expect a good to excellent outcome from lower extremity peripheral nerve decompression.

Discussion

These data confirm that compressive neuropathy of the upper extremity that presents as carpal tunnel syndrome, is the likely etiology behind neuropathy patients who are treated successfully with lower extremity nerve decompression. During the initial consultation with a patient who has diabetic neuropathy, it is important to learn if the patient has upper extremity peripheral nerve symptoms and if they had a previous decompression of the median nerve in the carpal tunnel. This study demonstrates that a good result from upper extremity peripheral nerve surgery predicts the outcome for lower extremity peripheral nerve surgery in 88% of patients, and is, therefore, information valuable for prognosis and clinical decision-making. These patients have a high probability of a successful outcome for restoration of sensation and relief of pain. In addition, this information can help surgeons decide appropriate candidates for lower extremity nerve decompression and help predict good outcomes.

References

[1] Boulton AJM, Malik RA. Diabetic neuropathy. Med Clin North Am 1998;82:909–29.
[2] Vinik AI. Diagnosis and management of diabetic neuropathy. Clin Geriatr Med 1999;15: 293.
[3] The Diabetes Control and Complications Trial Research Group. Factors in the development of diabetic neuropathy: baseline analysis of neuropathy in the feasibility phase of the Diabetes Control and Complications Trial (DCCT). Diabetes 1988;37:476.

[4] Maser RE, Steenkiste AR, Dorman JS, et al. Epidemiological correlates of diabetic report. Report from Pittsburgh Epidemiology of Diabetes Complications Study. Diabetes 1989;38: 1456–61.

[5] Dyck PJ, Dratz KM, Karnes JL, et al. The prevalence by staged severity of various types of diabetic neuropathy, retinopathy, and nephropathy in a population-based cohort: the Rochester Diabetic Neuropathy Study. Neurology 1993;43:817.

[6] Young MJ, Boulton AJM, Macleod AF, et al. A multicentre study of the prevalence of diabetic peripheral neuropathy in the United Kingdom hospital clinic population. Diabetologia 1993;36:150.

[7] Feldman EL, Stevens MJ, Thomas PK, et al. A practical two-step quantitative clinical and electrophysiological assessment for the diagnosis and staging of diabetic neuropathy. Diabetes Care 1994;17:1281.

[8] Federle D, Comi G, Coscelli C, et al. A multicenter study on the prevalence of diabetic neuropathy in Italy. Diabetes Care 1997;20:836.

[9] Sands ML, Shetterly SM, Franklin GM, et al. Incidence of distal symmetric (sensory) neuropathy in NIDDM. The San Luis Valley Diabetes Study. Diabetes Care 1997;20: 322.

[10] Cabezas-Cerrato J. The prevalence of clinical diabetic polyneuropathy in Spain: a study in primary care and hospital clinic groups. Diabetologia 1998;41:1263–9.

[11] DeWytt CN, Jackson RV, Hockings GI, et al. Polyneuropathy in Australian outpatients with type II diabetes mellitus. J Diabetes Complications 1999;13:74.

[12] Pirat J. Diabetes mellitus and its degenerative complications: a prospective study of 4,400 patients observed between 1947 and 1973. Diabetes Care 1978;1:168–88.

[13] Akbari CM, LoGerfo FW. The impact of micro- and macrovascular disease on diabetic neuropathy and foot problems. In: Veves A, editor. Clinical management of diabetic neuropathy. Totowa (NJ): Humana Press; 1998. p. 319–31.

[14] Palumbo JP, Melton LJ. Peripheral vascular disease and diabetes. In: Harris M, Jamman R, editors. Diabetes in America. Washington (DC): US Government Printing Office; 1985. p. XV. p. 1–21.

[15] Moss SE, Klein R, Kelin BEK. The prevalence and incidence of lower extremity amputation in a diabetic population. Arch Intern Med 1992;152:610–6.

[16] Resnick HE, Valsania P, Phillisps CL. Diabetes mellitus and nontraumatic lower extremity amputation in black and white Americans: The National Health and Nutrition Examination Survey Epidemiologic Follow-up Study 1971–1992. Arch Intern Med 1999;159:2470–5.

[17] Frykberg RG. Epidemiology of the diabetic foot: ulcerations and amputation. Adv Wound Care 1999;12:139.

[18] Diabetes Control and Complications Trial Research Group. The effect of intensive diabetes therapy on measures of autonomic nervous system function in the Diabetes Control and Complications Trial (DCCT). Diabetologia 1998;41:416–23.

[19] Cavanagh PR, Derr JA, Ulbrecht JS, et al. Problems with gait and posture in neuropathic patients with insulin-dependent diabetes mellitus. Diabet Med 1992;9:469–74.

[20] Simoneau GG, Ulbrecht JS, Derr JA, et al. Postural instability in patients with diabetic sensory neuropathy. Diabetes Care 1994;17:1411–21.

[21] Wallace C, Reiber GE, LeMaster J, et al. Incidence of falls, risk factors for falls, and fall-related fractures in individual with diabetes and a prior foot ulcer. Diabetes Care 2002;25: 1983.

[22] Cooner-Kerr T, Templeton MS. Chronic fall risk among aged individuals with type-2 diabetes. Ostomy Wound Manage 2002;48:28–34.

[23] Rull JA, Quibera R, Gonzalez-Millan H, et al. Symptomatic treatment of peripheral diabetic neuropathy with carbamazepine (Tegretol): double blind crossover trial. Diabetologia 1969; 5:215–8.

[24] Saudek CD, Werns S, Reidenberg MM. Phenytoin in the treatment of diabetic symmetrical polyneuropathy. Clin Pharmacol Ther 1977;22:196–9.

[25] Khurana RC. Treatment of painful diabetic neuropathy with trazadone. JAMA 1983;250: 1392.

[26] Kvinesdal B, Molin J, Froland A, et al. Imipramine treatment for painful diabetic neuropathy. JAMA 1984;251:1727–30.

[27] Morello CM, Leckband CG, Stoner CP, et al. Randomized double-blind study comparing the efficacy of gabapentin with amitriptyline on diabetic peripheral neuropathy pain. Arch Intern Med 1999;159:1931.

[28] Joss JD. Tricyclic antidepressant use in diabetic neuropathy. Ann Pharmacother 1999;33: 996–1000.

[29] Pecoraro RE, Reiber GE, Burgess EM. Pathways to diabetic limb amputation: basis for prevention. Diabetes Care 1990;13:513–21.

[30] Ollendorf D, Kotsanos J, Wishner W. Potential economic benefits of lower-extremity amputation prevention strategies in diabetes. Diabetes Care 1998;21:1240–5.

[31] Centers for Disease Control and Prevention. Diabetes surveillance, 1993. Atlanta (GA): US Department of Health and Human Services; 1993.

[32] Bloomgarden ZT. American Diabetres Association 60th Scientific Sessions, 2000: the diabetic foot. Diabetes Care 2001;24(5):946–51.

[33] Ramsey SD, Newton K, Blough D, et al. Incidence, outcomes, and cost of foot ulcers in patients with diabetes. Diabetes Care 1999;22:382–7.

[34] Gordois A, Oglesby A, Scuffham P, et al. The health care costs of diabetic peripheral neuropathy in the US. Diabetes Care 2003;26:1790–5.

[35] Harris MI, Flegal KM, Cowie CC, et al. Prevalence of diabetes, impaired fasting glucose, and impaired glucose tolerance in US adults: the Third National Health and Nutrition Examination Survey, 1988–1994. Diabetes Care 1998;21:518–24.

[36] Weinstock RS. Treating type 2 diabetes mellitus: a growing epidemic. Mayo Clin Proc 2003; 78:411–3.

[37] Hill JO. What to do about the metabolic syndrome? Arch Intern Med 2003;163:395–7.

[38] Bloombardern AT. Type 2 diabetes in the young: the evolving epidemic. Diabetes Care 2004; 27:998–1010.

[39] Centers for Disease Control and Prevention. History of foot ulcer among persons with diabetes–United States, 2000–2002. MMWR 2003;52(45):1098–102.

[40] Aszmann OC, Tassler PL, Dellon AL. Changing the natural history of diabetic neuropathy: incidence of ulcer/amputation in the contralateral limb of patients with a unilateral nerve decompression procedure. Ann Plast Surg 2004;53:517–22.

[41] Jakobsen J. Peripheral nerves in early experimental diabetes. Expansion of the endoneurial space as a cause of increased water content. Diabetologia 1978;14:113–9.

[42] Jakobsen J, Sidenius P. Decreased axonal transport of structural proteins in Streptozotocin diabetic rats. J Clin Invest 1980;66:292–1.

[43] Lundborg G, Rydevik B. Effects of stretching the tibial nerve of the rabbit, a preliminary study of the intraneural circulation and the barrier function of the perineurium. J Bone Joint Surg 1973;55B:390–401.

[44] Rydevik B, Lundborg G. Effects of graded compression on intraneural blood flow. J Hand Surg 1981;6A:3–12.

[45] Dellon AL, Mackinnon SE, Seiler WA. Susceptibility of the diabetic nerve to chronic compression. Ann Plast Surg 1988;20:117–9.

[46] Mackinnon SE, Dellon AL, Hudson AR, et al. Chronic nerve compression–an experimental model in the rat. Ann Plast Surg 1984;13:112–20.

[47] Ascherman JA, Knowles SL, Attkiss K. Docetaxel (Taxotere) extravasation: a report of five cases with treatment recommendations. Ann Plast Surg 2000;45:438–41.

[48] Langenstein HN, Duman H, Seelig D, et al. Retrospective study of the management of chemotherapeutic extravasation injury. Ann Plast Surg 2002;49:369.

[49] Thompson SW, Davis LE, Kornfeld M. Cisplatin neuropathy. Clinical, electrophysiologic, morphologic and toxicologic studies. Cancer 1984;54(7):1269–75.

[50] Cersosimo RJ. Cisplatin neurotoxicity. Cancer Treat Rev 1989;16(4):195–211.

[51] Mollman JE. Cisplatin neurotoxicity. N Engl J Med 1990;322:126–7.

[52] Rowinsky EK, Eisenhauer EA, Chaudhry V, et al. Clinical toxicities encountered with paclitaxel (Taxol). Semin Oncol 1993;20:1–15.

[53] Verweij J, Clavel M, Chevalier B. Paclitaxel (Taxol) and docetaxel (Taxotere): not simply two of a kind. Ann Oncol 1994;4:495–505.

[54] Pronk LC, Stoter G, Verweij J. Docetaxel (Taxotere): single agent activity, development of combination treatment and reducing side-effects. Cancer Treat Rev 1995;21:463–78.

[55] Dellon AL. Optimism in diabetic neuropathy. Ann Plast Surg 1988;20:103–5.

[56] Dellon AL, Mackinnon SE, Seiler WA IV. Susceptibility of the diabetic nerve to chronic compression. Ann Plast Surg 1988;20:117–9.

[57] Dellon ES, Dellon AL, Seiler WA IV. The effect of tarsal tunnel decompression in the streptozotocin-induced diabetic rat. Microsurgery 1994;15:265–8.

[58] Dellon AL. Treatment of symptoms of diabetic neuropathy by peripheral nerve decompression. Plast Reconstr Surg 1992;89:689–97.

[59] Wieman TJ, Patel VG. Treatment of hyperesthetic neuropathic pain in diabetics: decompression of the tarsal tunnel. Ann Surg 1995;221:660–5.

[60] Chafee H. Decompression of peripheral nerves for diabetic neuropathy. Plast Reconstr Surg 2000;106:813–5.

[61] Aszmann OA, Kress KM, Dellon AL. Results of decompression of peripheral nerves in diabetics: a prospective, blinded study. Plast Reconstr Surg 2000;106:816–21.

[62] Dellon AL. Prevention of foot ulcerations and amputation by decompression of peripheral nerve in patients with diabetic neuropathy. Ostomy Wound Manage 2002;48:36–45.

[63] Tassler PL, Dellon AL, Lesser GJ, et al. Utility of decompressive surgery in the prophylaxis and treatment of cisplatin neuropathy in adult rats. J Reconstr Microsurg 2000;16:457.

[64] Dellon AL, Swier P, Maloney CT, et al. Chemotherapy-induced neuropathy: treatment by decompression of peripheral nerves. Plast Reconstr Surg 2004;114(2):478–83.

[65] Perkins BA, Olaaleye D, Bril V. Carpal tunnel syndrome in patients with diabetic polyneuropathy. Diabetes Care 2002;25:565–74.

[66] Mackinnon SE, Dellon AL. Surgery of the peripheral nerve. New York: Thieme Publishing; 1988.

[67] Dellon AL. Operative technique for submuscular transposition of the ulnar nerve. Contemp Orthop 1988;16:17–24.

[68] Dellon AL. Techniques for successful management of ulnar nerve entrapment at the elbow. Neurosurg Clin N Am 1991;2:57–73.

[69] Dellon AL, Mackinnon SE. Radial sensory nerve entrapment in the forearm. J Hand Surg 1986;11A:199–205.

[70] Mont MA, Dellon AL, Chen F, et al. Operative treatment of peroneal nerve palsy. J Bone Joint Surg 1996;78A:863–9.

[71] Dellon AL. Entrapment of the deep peroneal nerve on the dorsum of the foot. Foot Ankle 1990;11:73–80.

[72] Keck C. The tarsal tunnel syndrome. J Bone Joint Surg 1962;44A:180–8.

[73] Lam SJS. A tarsal tunnel syndrome. Lancet 1962;2:1354–5.

[74] Mackinnon SE, Dellon AL. Homologies between the tarsal and carpal tunnels: implications for treatment of the tarsal tunnel syndrome. Contemp Orthop 1987;14:75–9.

[75] Dellon AL. Computer-assisted sensibility evaluation and surgical treatment of tarsal tunnel syndrome. Adv Podiatry 1996;2:17–40.

[76] Dellon AL. Tinel or not tinel. J Hand Surg 1984;9B:216.

ELSEVIER
SAUNDERS

Clin Podiatr Med Surg
23 (2006) 569–578

CLINICS IN
PODIATRIC
MEDICINE AND
SURGERY

Intermetatarsal Compression Neuritis

Justin Franson, DPM, Babak Baravarian, DPM*

*Foot and Ankle Institute, 2121 Wilshire Boulevard,
Suite 101, Santa Monica, CA 90403, USA*

Intermetatarsal neuroma has been well described in the literature over the years. Although the condition often bears the name of Morton, who described the condition in 1876 [1], the original description has been attributed to Durlacher in 1845 [2].

"Morton's neuroma" is not a true neuroma, although the use of the term has been perpetuated in the literature. A more accurate description of this condition is intermetatarsal compression neuritis (ICN), which will be used in this article. This forefoot pathology can be a disabling condition; individuals who don't respond well to initial treatments are left with persistent pain and frustration. The treatment options have evolved over the years and there are now more options available to the practitioner than the simple conservative treatments and surgical resection. It is important to understand the condition well, and pursue new treatment protocols that can lead to improved outcomes.

Occurrence

Although the condition can be found in any individual, ICN is more common in middle-aged females, especially those who frequently wear high-heeled and pointed-toe shoes [3]. The abnormal biomechanical forces and toe crowding caused by many fashionable shoes have been suggested as etiological factors in the development of this condition.

It is generally accepted that the third intermetatarsal space is the anatomic location most susceptible to ICN [3]. Dockery [4] reported results on 100 neuromas, of which 81 cases involved the third intermetatarsal space. However, in one long-term follow-up study of ICN, 67% of 70 neuromas treated were located in the second intermetatarsal space [5]. First and fourth interspace neuromas are rare [3].

---

* Corresponding author.

E-mail address: bbaravarian@mednet.ucla.edu (B. Baravarian).

0891-8422/06/$ - see front matter © 2006 Elsevier Inc. All rights reserved.
doi:10.1016/j.cpm.2006.04.002   *podiatric.theclinics.com*

Anatomy

The intermetatarsal nerves that pass between the metatarsal heads are branches from the medial and lateral plantar nerves, the continuation of the tibial nerve. The third intermetatarsal space receives nerve contributions from a branch of the medial and lateral plantar nerves. It has been suggested that the nerve is larger in this area because of the two nerve branches that join here, which provides an anatomic explanation for the more common occurrence of neuroma in the third intermetatarsal space. Furthermore, there is a noted medial and lateral column to the foot where the third metatarsal is connected to a stable cuneiform; the fourth metatarsal is connected to a more mobile cubiod. This may facilitate greater motion at the third interspace level between the metatarsal heads, which results in nerve irritation and fibrosis.

As they near the distal level of the metatarsals, the common digital nerves pass beneath, or plantar to, the deep transverse intermetatarsal ligament. The nerves then branch into the proper plantar digital nerves, and supply sensory innervation to the toes.

Etiology

Although there has been some difference of opinon regarding the pathoetiology of this condition, it is frequently attributed to a mechanical entrapment neuropathy as the nerves pass between the metatarsal heads. It has been suggested that the histopathologic appearance of neuromas are related to two types of microtrauma: stretching and compression [6].

Intermetatarsal compression neuritis can occur in a pronated, supinated, or neutral foot. In the Cavus foot type, it has been suggested that there is increased tension on the plantar fascia and the deep transverse intermetatarsal ligament [7]. This tension in the deep fascia structures render them less forgiving and place a more rigid structure under which the nerve will pass. When the toes are placed in a relative dorsiflexed position by highheeled shoes, or as they dorsiflex in the propulsive phase of the gait cycle, the intermetatarsal nerves are placed against the tight, deep transverse metatarsal ligament. Routine radiographs obtained in the work-up of ICN in relation to cavus feet often shows a relative proximity of the metatarsal heads in the affected intermetatarsal space.

Pronated and neutral feet may also be affected with ICN. The authors have observed that in neutral or pronated feet, there is often hypermotion of the metatarsal heads (noted as "a loose bag of bones") that results in excess compression and motion at the metatarsal heads and neuritis or fibrosis of the nerve.

Diagnosis

A careful review of the patient's description of the symptoms coupled with a physical examination will usually be sufficient to arrive at the diagnosis of neuroma. Symptoms can include pain at the ball of the foot, burning pain, tingling, numbness in the toes, pain radiating into the toes or proximally into the arch, cramping, a shooting or stabbing pain, or a feeling like the patient is walking on a pebble or knot. Neuromas are not always easy to distinguish from other conditions that affect this anatomic area of the foot. Differential diagnosis can include tarsal tunnel syndrome or peripheral neuropathy, metatarsal stress fracture, tear of the plantar plate, plantar metatarsophalangeal joint capsulitis, avascular necrosis of the metatarsal head, metatarsal bone tumor, soft tissue mass, bursitis, flexor digitorum tendonitis, and hammertoes that cause a retrograde buckling force and induce metatarsalgia.

Physical examination includes direct, deep palpation of the intermetatarsal space. Pain can usually be induced with deep intermetatarsal palpation, and simultaneous side-to-side compression of the metatarsals. This will often produce the "Mulder's sign," a palpable and sometimes audible click of the neuroma between the metatarsal heads. Diagnostic injections at the distal intermetatarsal space using a local anesthetic can help differentiate the distal ICN from a more proximal cause, such as tarsal tunnel syndrome or peripheral neuropathy.

Pressure specified sensory testing (PSSD) is a newer diagnostic tool which can be used to help rule out the presence of tarsal tunnel or other peripheral compression neuropathy. It can be used to evaluate and confirm an ICN, however, it is more difficult to examine the lesser digital nerve function. A more complete discussion of PSSD testing is given in the neurosensory testing article by Soomekh and colleagues elsewhere in this issue.

Imaging

Evaluation of ICN will often lead to routine radiographs, which can help rule-out other pathology. It is common to see a relative closer proximity of the adjacent metatarsal heads in the affected intermetatarsal space.

Although the diagnosis of ICN is largely based on clinical suspicion after a review of the patient's symptomatology and a thorough clinical examination, imaging is sometimes used pre-operatively. There can, however, be false negatives and false positives that may confuse the decision-making progress. The use of computerized tomography, diagnostic ultrasound, and MRI have been presented in the literature [8–10] as acceptable forms of imaging that can yield relatively accurate images of the affected nerve, although in most cases, they are used to rule out other possible causes of pain and symptoms. To complicate diagnosis, ICN does not always produce the bulbous swelling and nerve enlargement sometimes seen with this condition.

Ultrasound can be a very reliable modality to detect the pathology. This does rely, however, on an experienced ultrasonographer as well as a high-quality device. Ultrasound is less expensive than MRI or CT, and does not expose the patient to radiation. The procedure is performed by placing the probe parallel and just distal to the metatarsal heads. The potential involved interspace is then pressed from a dorsal motion and an enlarged nerve branch may be noted plantar to the transverse intermetatarsal ligament. A second position is to place the probe in a linear fashion, dorsally between the metatarsal heads, and observe the nerve in a longitudinal fashion. This is far more difficult to perform and requires a highly skilled ultrasonographer.

Multiple papers have discussed ultrasound diagnosis of ICN in the foot. A paper by Mendicino and colleagues [9] reported accurate detection of the presence, location, and size of the neuroma, as high as 95%–98%. However, in another study that compared pre-operative imaging with surgical findings, approximately half of the neuromas were missed by ultrasound and MRI [11].

Magnetic resonance imaging can produce the finest soft-tissue contrast. The edematous nerve is best seen on a T1-weighted image, and will be visualized as a localized mass with lower signal intensity. However, the edematous region can also be missed if the slices of imaging are not close enough together and the region is not filmed properly.

Pathology

Differing information exists in the literature regarding the pathologic findings in the presence of symptomatic neuromas.

In a 2000 study by Morscher and colleagues [12], the morphology and histological findings of ICN were checked. The excised neuromas were compared with biopsies of similar cadaver intermetatarsal nerves. They found no qualitative differences in the histomorphological examination of neuromas as compared with the cadaver specimens. The study did observe differences in the nerve diameter, although increased diameter is not always seen. This study further showed that the 17 smallest diameter nerves they examined were from autopsy specimens, and the 5 largest diameter nerves were from resected neuromas. The medium diameter nerves showed a wide overlap of the neuroma and the normal cadaver specimens. Based on this information, they concluded that MRI and ultrasonography are not necessary when deciding about surgical intervention, and were less reliable than diagnostic local anesthetic injections [12].

The only problem with local injections, is differentiation of plantar plate tears from neuroma pain, because both will improve with injection. However, with proper clinical correlation, a differentiation may be made.

Conservative treatment

The conservative approach to the treatment of neuromas includes shoe modifications, padding, orthotics, cortisone injections, and serial alcohol sclerosing injections [8]. The response to the conservative treatment of

ICN is often directly related to the persistence, focused treatment, and creativity of physician. Those who more aggressively use the conservative measures are more likely to alleviate pain without surgical intervention. An article in *Foot and Ankle International* [6] concluded that orthotics that control rearfoot pronation produced no significant benefit in treating this condition.

It is well known that ICN is more commonly found in females, often middle-aged women. Shoes have been implicated as a causative factor in the development of neuromas. Shoe modifications should be strongly encouraged: wide toe box shoes and flat, heel-less shoes are best.

Cortisone injections are a well-accepted conservative treatment of the symptoms of neuroma, although they will likely not have a lasting effect unless other modifications are instituted. The injected steroid provides an anti-inflammatory mechanism at the area of pathology.

A series of dilute alcohol slerosing injections has been proposed as a favorable conservative treatment. The injected solution, a dehydrated alcohol mixed with local anesthetic with epinephrine, has a high affinity for nerve tissue, and produces a chemical neurolysis. Dockery's [8] paper reported that 89% of patients improved. Long-term outcomes with this treatment have yet to be presented. The authors have been unable to reproduce such a high rate of success using the alcohol sclerosing injections. In spite of this, it is a useful option, especially for patients who are not surgical candidates, or prefer to avoid surgical intervention.

Custom orthotics has been a standard treatment option for intermetatarsal neuritis. Although the effectiveness of this treatment has been questioned in the literature [6], the authors' clinical experience has been that orthotics can be helpful. By controlling the rearfoot and midtarsal joints, abnormal forefoot compensation can be alleviated. Placement of padding can also function to spread the metatarsals and cushion the ball of the foot.

Surgical treatment

When a person has failed conservative treatment for a forefoot neuroma, surgery can be considered to alleviate pain and treat the condition. Several different surgical approaches have been described in the literature.

Neurectomy

The traditional surgical approach has been to perform a surgical excision of the affected nerve proximal to the metatarsal heads. This can be accomplished using multiple incisional approaches: dorsal longitudinal, plantar transverse, and plantar longitudinal. The excision of the nerve has produced varied results. One study observed a 93% patient satisfaction rate over the long-term (average 4.8 years), after dorsal longitudinal incision was used for neuroma excision [5]. The downside to performing nerve excision is the postoperative dysesthesias and the potential for a painful stump neuroma.

Carbon dioxide laser

A study by Wasserman [13] discussed the use and clinical outcome of a carbon dioxide laser in neuroma therapy. The author relates excellent results; of 50 randomly sampled cases, there was only a single complication, and that was related to use of the ankle tourniquet. One noted benefit of the laser was that the nerve stump was sealed. Their patients were able to return to normal ambulation faster than with the conventional surgical approach.

Neurolysis

Another surgical approach is to perform a neurolysis, or surgical nerve decompression. This can be done endoscopically or through an open approach. The authors' preference is through an open approach, so they can directly see the area (Figs. 1 and 2). This also facilitates opening the endoneurium. The procedure is performed through a 2–3 cm dorsally based incision, placed in the noted interspace. Blunt dissection is carried to the level of the intermetatarsal ligament and a freer elevator or straight hemostat is placed plantar to the ligament (Fig. 3). The ligament is then linearly incised and cauterized at the edges with a bipolar style cautery to prevent damage to the nerve. Any scar and fibrosis about the nerve is then released under high-power magnification (Fig. 4). Suturing the skin is performed with the surgeon's choice of closure. On the day of surgery the patient is allowed to apply weight in a surgical shoe and can move into a tennis shoe at 1 week when wound healing has progressed. Physical therapy is started at 2 weeks to break up fibrosis.

A recent article discussed intermetatarsal nerve decompression with relocation dorsal to the intermetatarsal ligament of the digital nerve [14]. The article presented the surgical outcomes of 82 feet, 95% of which had complete resolution of neuritic symptoms within an average of 7 days following surgery.

Review of neurolysis results

The Foot and Ankle Institute Network has followed the progress of the authors' first 30 cases of intermetatarsal nerve decompression over the past year. The procedure is performed through a linear interspace incision for each involved interspace. The incision is deepened and the intermetatarsal ligament is released. Careful dissection of the nerve is then performed; any fibrosis about the nerve is debrided, and the nerve is decompressed as needed under visualization with high-power magnification loupes.

The overall findings have been excellent: pain relief resulted in all cases. Three 3 of the 30 cases have had some level of continued pain after neurolysis. One case had previous alcohol injections for three sessions before neurolysis; a neurectomy was eventually performed because the nerve pain

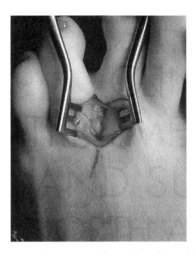

Fig. 1. Neuroma 1. Intermetatarsal neuroma with noted swelling of the nerve distal to the compression site of the intermetatarsal ligament and metatarsal heads.

did not resolve completely following decompression. A second case had no pain but felt mild tenderness and discomfort from the enlarged nerve "popping" against the metatarsal head region. This resolved with time and an orthotic device and no further surgery or treatment was deemed necessary. A third case with post-operative pain was noted to have symptoms consistent with complex regional pain syndrome. Conservative management of this patient has resulted in gradual improvement of symptoms, and a return to normal activities.

Two cases treated with previous alcohol injection from other physicians were treated with decompression. Resolution of pain and tingling to the toes was noted following decompression, which was not found with the alcohol treatments.

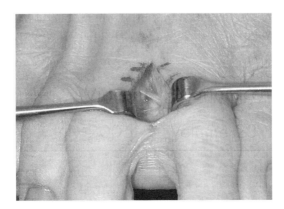

Fig. 2. Neuroma Pre-1. Fibrous band and intersmetatarsal ligament before decompression.

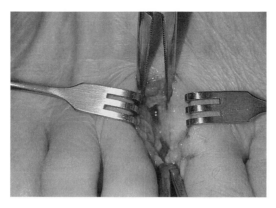

Fig. 3. Neuroma Pre-2. Hemostat placed plantar to the intermetatarsal ligament before release.

Overall satisfaction rate has been 90%; there were no major complications and no gross long-term pain or loss of function. One finding is that it is essential to return the patient to a flexible shoe as soon as incision healing is noted. This will facilitate movement of the nerve and less scarring. This should also be combined with physical therapy to break up further scaring. A second finding is that the alcohol treatments may resolve localized nerve entrapment, but the more proximal nerve tissue may still be compressed which results in pain that may be helped by decompression.

Treatment of recurrent or stump neuromas

Wolfort and Dellon [15] have described their surgical technique for nerve resection through a plantar approach: they implant the proximal end of the nerve into the muscle belly. They have reported that with this approach, 80% of patients had excellent relief from symptoms. The authors' current

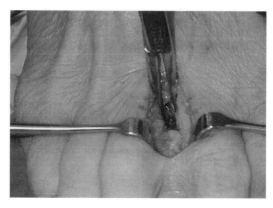

Fig. 4. Neuroma Post-1. Intermetatarsal nerve following decompression of the intermetatarsal ligament.

treatment of stump neuromas depends on the site of the stump neuroma and whether the stump neuroma involves one or two interspaces. If one interspace stump is involved, a linear plantar incision is made in the central metatarsal region but in the associated interspace. The neuroma is identified proximal to the stump site and buried into the arch region, into a deep muscle or local metatarsal. It is essential to bury the muscle away from a weight-bearing surface and in a region of little to no movement. Therefore, the lumbrical muscle belly, the quadratus plantae, and the metatarsal region are the best noted sites.

If two interspaces are involved, an incision is made over the metatarsal that divides the two interspaces to give access to both interspaces. Again, the incision is in the arch region and away from the metatarsal head region or interspace region.

Using this current technique, the authors have performed a series of 12 cases in the past 2 years. These cases have all been associated with previous neuroma surgery for point tenderness associated with stump neuroma. One case involved the second and third interspace; the other 11 cases involved the third interspace only. All cases required dissection of the nerve into the arch region and burial into a deep muscle. No bone burial was performed. The nerve was not sutured into the muscle belly but was turned proximally and buried about 1 cm into the belly of a deep arch muscle. All cases responded to treatment: 3 cases reported mild pain and 9 cases reported no pain. No scar formation was noted and no patient stated that they would not have done the surgery again. No patient required pain medication following surgery. Three patients experienced pain. One was associated with peripheral neuropathy and two cases were associated with previous diagnosis of reflex sympathetic dystrophy.

Summary

It is somewhat disturbing to consider that nerve resection is performed as a primary procedure only on the foot and not in any other region of the body. The thinking behind this type of surgery has been that there is severe damage to the nerve itself, which leads to scarring of the nerve fibers. As a result, the nerve is removed or resected in its scar portion. However, microscopic observation of the nerve shows that there may be surrounding nerve fibrosis and edema of the actual nerve, but the nerve itself is actually not damaged in its internal structure and the fascicles are stable. With this in mind, resection of the nerve seems to be a possible cause of stump pain and may not be the best primary option.

The authors find that in most of their cases, the nerve is compressed by the intermetatarsal ligament, and that there is edema of the nerve distal to the ligament and no alteration of the nerve proximal to the ligament site. This would then mean that the edema may be from a compression and not from an internal derangement.

As a result of our findings, a protocol is followed at The Foot and Ankle Institute Network. Following a period of conservative care, if there is still pain, a decompression of the interspace is considered. This is done with an open procedure to facilitate neurolysis of the nerve if needed. In cases of poor surgical candidates or in those who select a more non-invasive approach, alcohol injections may be attempted. In both cases, it is explained that there may be a need for nerve resection if there is continued pain and if the surgery is not successful. However, the results to date show that decompression is similar to neurectomy surgery, if not more successful.

References

[1] Morton TG. A peculiar and painful affection of the fourth metatarsophalangeal articulation. Am J Med Sci 1876;71:37–45.

[2] Durlacher L. A treatise on corns, bunions, the disease of nails, and the general management of the feet. London: Simkin, Marshall & Co.; 1845.

[3] Wu KK. Morton's interdigital neuroma: a clinical review of its etiology, treatment, and results. J Foot Ankle Surg 1996;35(2):112–9.

[4] Dockery GL. The treatment of intermetatarsal neuromas with 4% alcohol sclerosing injections. J Foot Ankle Surg 1999;38(6):403–8.

[5] Keh RA, Ballew KK, Higgins KR, et al. Long-term follow-up of Morton's neuroma. J Foot Surg 1992;31(1):93–5.

[6] Kilmartin TE, Wallace WA. Effect of pronation and supination orthosis on Morton's neuroma and lower extremity function. Foot Ankle Int 1994;15(5):256–62.

[7] Wachter SD, Nilson RZ, Thul JR. The relationship between foot structure and intermetatarsal neuromas. J Foot Surg 1984;23:436–9.

[8] Biasca N, Zanetti M, Zollinger H. Outcomes after partial neurectomy of Morton's neuroma related to preoperative case histories, clinical findings, and findings on magneticv resonance imaging. Foot Ankle Int 1999;20(9):568–75.

[9] Mendicino SS, Rockett MS. Morton's neuroma, update on diagnosis and imaging. Clin Podiatr Med Surg 1997;14(2):303–11.

[10] Sharp RJ, Wade CM, Hennessy MS, et al. The role of MRI and ultrasound imaging in Morton's neuroma and the effect of size of lesion on symptoms. J Bone Joint Surg 2003; 85-B(7):999–1005.

[11] Resch S, Stenstrom A, Jonsson A, et al. The diagnostic efficacy of magnetic resonance imaging and ultrasonography in Morton's neuroma: a radiologic-surgical correlation. Foot Ankle 1994;15(2):88–92.

[12] Morscher E, Ulrich J, Dick W. Morton's intermetatarsal neuroma: morphology and histological substrate. Foot Ankle Int 2000;21(7):558–62.

[13] Wasserman G. Treatment of Morton's neuroma with the carbon dioxide laser. Clin Podiatr Med Surg 1992;9(3):671–86.

[14] Vito GR, Talarico LM. A modified technique for Morton's neuroma. Decompression with relocation. J Am Podiatr Med Assoc 2003;93(3):190–4.

[15] Wolfort SF, Dellon AL. Treatment of recurrent neuroma of the interdigital nerve by implantation of the proximal nerve into muscle in the arch of the foot. J Foot Ankle Surg 2001;40(6):404–10.

ELSEVIER
SAUNDERS

Clin Podiatr Med Surg
23 (2006) 579–595

CLINICS IN
PODIATRIC
MEDICINE AND
SURGERY

Endoscopic Nerve Decompression

Stephen L. Barrett, DPM, MBA, CWS

*Arizona Podiatric Medicine Program, Midwestern University, College of Health Sciences,
19555 North 59th Avenue, Glendale, AZ 85308, USA*

Over the past decade there has been movement in all surgical specialties toward less-invasive surgery. It has been well documented that patients who undergo endoscopic or minimally invasive procedures usually have less pain and postoperative morbidity, and an earlier return to regular activity when compared with those who have had "open" procedures for the same condition [1,2].

In order for one to gain a clearer perspective, and more informed assessment of newer, less-invasive surgical modalities it helps to have an idea of how past history has shaped future development.

History of Morton's Neuroma

This is especially true in the treatment of Morton's entrapment, and other forefoot nerve entrapments. Nomenclature of a disease or condition can affect types and choices of a surgical approach or technique. Morton's neuroma is a misnomer, and unfortunately surgical resection of the common plantar digital nerve (intermetatarsal nerve) has been long established as "standard of care" since Professor Hoadley in Chicago first described resection of the nerve for treatment of metatarsalgia in 1893 [3]. Clearly, the misnaming of this common forefoot nerve entrapment conveys misunderstanding of the etiology, and has lead to confusion among different medical specialties and factions, perpetuating the advocating of surgical resection versus decompression. There is still widespread belief within the universe of clinicians dedicated to foot and ankle surgery that the term "Morton's Neuroma" is long standing in the medical literature. This is not the case.

The author is a paid medical consultant for Instratek, Inc, Houston, TX, which manufactures the endoscopic instrumentation referenced in this article, and is also a shareholder in Sensory Management Services, which manufactures the PSSD neurosensory testing device that is also referenced in the article.

E-mail address: sbarre@midwestern.edu

The first documentation in the medical literature where the term "Morton's Neuroma" was used dates to only 1972 [4,5]. One must question why the erroneous term of "neuroma" was ever applied to the condition, and even more so readily adopted by the large body of clinicians, when similar pathophysiology and understanding of nerve compression syndromes in the hand and upper extremity were well described in the literature decades before 1972 [6]. There is even additional confusion of why the condition was attributed to Morton in the first place, aside from ignorance of foreign literature. Civininni [7] was the first to accurately document the symptom complex in 1835, which was some 41 years before the description of Thomas Morton in 1876 [8]. Between this time, Durlacher [9] and a citation of Heuter by Vogel [10] published their separate clinical findings, but yet their names were not included in the nomenclature. Additionally, there is more historical confusion, as there was a second Morton, a T.S.K. Morton who published about the same forefoot condition [11].

Etiology/pathophysiology of Morton's entrapment

The histological response to nerve compression is consistent regardless of the anatomical location of the entrapped peripheral nerve [12]. Characteristic microscopic findings associated with human chronic nerve compression include endoneurial and subepineurial edema as a result of disruption of the blood-nerve barrier, increased deposition of collagen within the connective tissues resulting in increased thickness or fibrosis of the perineurium and epineurium, and focal demylineation [12]. MacKinnon and Dellon [12] also pointed out that proximal and distal to the site of chronic nerve compression the neuron appears normal, both with the naked eye and microscopically. An interesting histopathological study was performed by Morscher and colleagues [13], where they demonstrated no histological difference between nerves that were resected for treatment of Morton's entrapment, and those resected from cadavers who had no history of metatarsalgia. They found epineurial and perineural fibrosis, a reduction in myelinated fibers, and hyalinization of endoneurial tissue. Graham and Graham, in 1984, concluded that the condition simply was a result of compression based on their histological findings [14]. Electron microscopic findings also lead Shereff and Grande [15] to conclude that Morton's disease was a result of localized impingement.

In light of the fact that there is overwhelming, objective scientific evidence that Morton's disease is a true entrapment, it is difficult to understand the reasoning and physiological basis for certain treatments that are currently being purported. These would include alcohol sclerosing injections, percutaneous electrocoagulation, radiofrequency destruction, and cryoablation [16–19].

Aside from the isolated patient who may be unable to undergo a surgical procedure, there is little scientific basis for destruction of a peripheral nerve that is simply entrapped. It is well documented that peripheral nerves that have been decompressed have the ability to regenerate after the source of compression is eliminated with neurolysis/decompression [20–22]. It is also well established that regardless of the modality involved in the resection of a peripheral nerve, true neuroma formation is a physiologic certainty. MacKinnon and Dellon [12] indicate that up to 150 different modalities have been described in the literature aimed to prevent the formation of neuroma after transection of a peripheral nerve. Clearly, with so many different approaches with very limited reported success, this is a strong statement about the seriousness of the complications that can result from transecting a peripheral nerve for the treatment of Morton's entrapment.

Nerve injury has been well categorized by histological and clinical criteria. Dellon delineates the different types of peripheral nerve injury in his text *Somatosensory Testing and Rehabilitation* [23] (see Table 1). Cryoablation, sclerosing injections, and destruction by electrical current or radiofrequency will cause some type of peripheral nerve injury. Caporusso and colleagues [16] reported treatment of 31 "neuromas" in 20 patients; however, there is confusion of what they are actually defining as a neuroma, as they included in their study patients who had "neuromas" of the sural and intermediate dorsal cutaneous nerves as well as those in the intermetatarsal spaces. In their article, they claim to locate the nerve by a nerve stimulator, which elicits a pain response when the nerve is close to the tip of the cryoprobe. The accuracy of their percutaneous method must be questioned in response to their own poor reported results. Only 38.7% of their patients were completely pain free at 1 year, while 45.2% reported some improvement in pain, with 16.1% having no improvement. Interestingly, research on the palmar and plantar digital nerves in the horse led to the conclusion that a percutaneous technique caused a temporary loss of pain perception that only lasted for a few weeks [24]. These same authors documented histology of "neuromas in continuity," a type VI nerve injury in 10 of the 28 specimens harvested after the horses were euthanized. A recent report on the treatment of upper extremity nerve injuries with cryotherapy, however, showed promising results, but emphasized that the nerve must actually be surgically exposed before freezing [25]. Another

Table 1
Classification of nerve injury

Type of injury	Description	Recovery
I Neuropraxia	Local conduction block	Complete
II Axontomesis	Axonal damage, but epineurium and perineurium are still intact	Complete
III Third degree	Scarring within endoneurium	Incomplete
IV Fourth degree	Physical continuity but not functioning	No recovery
V Neurotmesis	Nerve is transected in open injury	None without repair
VI Neuroma in continuity	Mixed fascicular damage	Possible partial

Courtesy of A. Lee Dellon, MD, Baltimore, Maryland.

distinction between their work and that of Caporusso and coworkers is that they were treating injured upper extremity peripheral nerves, and not entrapped peripheral nerves. In fact, in the Caporusso and colleagues' study [16], they report that all five of their patients who had no relief of pain had previous neurectomies. Based on these results, procedures oriented toward injury or resection of the peripheral nerve should be avoided, even if they are percutaneous and "nonsurgical."

Preoperative clinical evaluation and diagnosis of forefoot peripheral nerve entrapments

Many times when a given pathology is extremely common, it becomes easy for the clinician to sometimes jump to diagnostic conclusions, only to find out later that after some type of intervention has occurred, there is additional or other pathology that is really responsible for the patient's symptoms. This is frequently the case with Morton's entrapment, of which the diagnosis is most commonly made by history and clinical examination alone [26]. The clinical examination often times only consists of simple palpation, and maybe a plain dorsal-plantar radiograph. Mulder's sign is described as a clicking, with palpation in the interspace when the forefoot is compressed from medial to lateral [27]. The author has been able to elicit a positive Mulder's sign on patients with no complaints of forefoot nerve entrapment, and one must question the hanging a complete diagnosis solely on the presence of this sign. Another sign that may be useful, but is subjected to wide levels of interpretation, is if there is pain with palpation of the interspace, with accompanying radiation or a "shooting" sensation distally or proximally. The clinician should also palpate the adjacent metatarsalphalangeal joints to ascertain that the patient is not suffering from a capsulitis, rupture of the plantar plate, or an intra-articular derangement of the joint itself rather than a provocation sign of nerve entrapment.

As with all types of peripheral nerve pathology, patients will use different words and phraseology to describe their symptoms. Words like "shooting," "burning," and "sharp" are frequent. They may say that something just feels "like a sock is rolled up under my foot." Others will state they "have a feeling of pressure." It is important to ascertain how long the condition has been present, how has it been treated previously, if at all, and if changes in shoe gear make any difference.

Diagnostic tests

Numerous studies have advocated the use of diagnostic ultrasound for preoperative evaluation of a patient with Morton's symptoms [28–36]. It is likely that diagnostic musculoskeletal ultrasound is more useful in the diagnosis of Morton's entrapment for what it does not show. A complete forefoot examination with diagnostic ultrasound would rule out any capsular involvement, including rupture of the plantar plates, and space-occupying lesions within the interspace, such as the frequently described "bursa." It is very common to see disruption of the plantar plate, with associated medial or lateral deviation of the digit, in patients who have been frequently injected with steroids, and also occasionally seen in the patient who has had percutaneous cyrotherapy (see Fig. 1 and Fig. 2). Also, there is a vast difference in the quality of diagnostic ultrasound machines out in the clinical setting. To adequately visualize the common plantar digital nerve, which is very superficial, requires a minimum of a 12 to 15 MHz high-frequency broadband linear array transducer [37]. Because of the sophisticated requirements of both the user's skill and interpretive ability, as well as the machine, visualization can sometimes be difficult. It is not uncommon that when some clinicians are attempting visualization of a peripheral nerve such as the common plantar digital (intermetatarsal), which is of a small diameter, they purport that there is evidence of a large neuromatous mass, which in reality is sonographic artifact.

Magnetic resonance imaging (MRI) has also been suggested as a useful diagnostic tool in helping differentiate other forefoot pathology from Morton's entrapment [38–40]. Two disadvantages of MRIs are that they are expensive, and the technology does not allow for a dynamic examination by the treating clinician.

Another useful diagnostic test before intervening with surgery for Morton's entrapment is the use of simple local anesthetic peripheral nerve blocks [41]. These can help differentiate adjacent interspace lesions in the patient

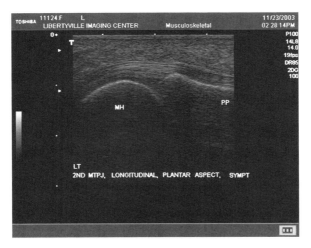

Fig. 1. In this high-resolution diagnostic ultrasound photo the plantar plate is visualized to be intact, of normal thickness, and to have normal signal intensity. (Courtesy of Brian Kincaid, Chicago, IL.)

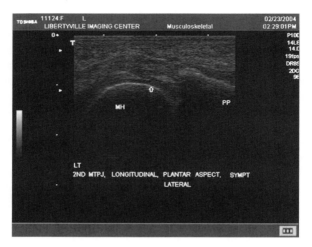

Fig. 2. This is the same patient as in Fig. 1, 3 months later, with a demonstrable plantar plate rupture resulting from sclerosing injections. (Courtesy of Brian Kincaid, Chicago, IL.)

with diffuse symptomatology, and can be highly predictive regarding potential outcome from neurolysis/decompression [42]. However, a positive clinical result from a small infiltration of a local anesthetic agent is not a good predictor if the nerve is denervated. The clinician must be sure to only infiltrate a small amount, usually less than 1 cc, only in the suspected interspace, so that anesthetic does not seep out peripherally, and block other potentially etiologic neural tissue.

Physical examination has always been the mainstay for diagnosis of forefoot peripheral nerve entrapments, but it is imperative to also evaluate proximally at the level of the tarsal tunnel. Any pain with gentle palpation on the Tibial nerve, or a positive Tinel's sign should caution the practitioner to rule out other nerve entrapments. Dellon [43] illustrated how common coexistent tarsal tunnel syndrome is with recurrent Morton's neuroma. He found a 75% incidence of entrapment at the level of the medial ankle in his series of patients. This should serve as a warning sign to any practitioner who sees the patient with multiple interspace involvement, unilaterally or bilaterally, that other proximal nerve entrapment may be at play. Jacoby [44] recently reported at the Institute for Peripheral Nerve Surgery's 2004 annual meeting that Morton's entrapment can be a very early marker for diabetes, or pre-diabetes (sometimes referred to as Syndrome X or metabolic disease). If there is any suspicion of proximal nerve involvement from either the focused clinical examination, or from a diffuse or nebulous history from the patient, it is warranted to obtain neurosensory testing with the PSSD (pressure specified sensory device) manufactured by Sensory Management Services, Baltimore, MD (see Fig. 3A–C). If there is additional nerve entrapment discovered, then the treating physician must make the decision to decompress the appropriate nerves involved.

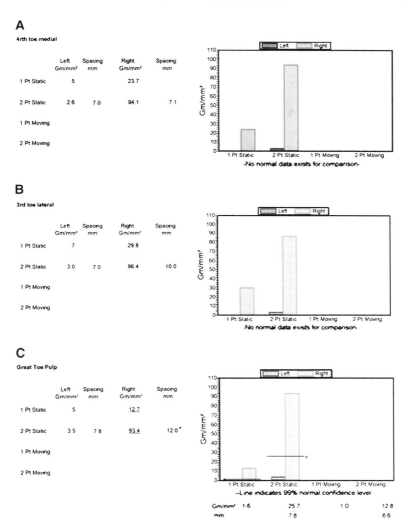

Fig. 3. (A–C) These are example neurosensory testing reports that demonstrate increased pressure thresholds for the medial plantar nerve of the right foot, which would indicate proximal entrapment at the level of the tarsal tunnel, as well as increased pressure thresholds for the affected quadrants of the third interspace. This report illustrates what is commonly seen in patients with "diffuse or nebulous" forefoot symptoms, which is oftentimes diagnosed as solely a Morton's entrapment.

This is especially true with the situation of adjacent interspace nerve entrapment. With procedures that rely on excision of the nerve, with a maximally traumatic open exposure, the surgeon oftentimes is reluctant to operate on adjacent interspaces simultaneously. This has not been the experience with endoscopic decompression by the author. There has never been a documented vascular embarrassment with concurrent adjacent interspace endoscopic decompressions, with the endoscopic decompression of intermetatarsal nerve (EDIN) system, and if performed judiciously there should be no cause to avoid decompressing both sites of entrapment.

Also in the preoperative work-up, the patient must be evaluated for the presence of Equinus, which is documented to be the etiological agent in most forefoot pathology, as well as being responsible for increased plantar forefoot pressures [45–48]. We recently reported a case of multiple interspace nerve entrapment, where there was diffuse forefoot pain, with additional isolated intermetatarsal nerve compression, associated with severe gastrocnemius equinus. The patient's forefoot symptoms were completely alleviated with endoscopic gastrocnemius recession, which increased dorsiflexion by 20 degrees, and decreased the maximal forefoot pressure, as measured by the F-scan from 39 psi to 19 psi for a 49% reduction in pressure [49].

There is still controversy and debate about frequency of forefoot nerve entrapment in other interspaces. By definition, Morton's entrapment can only exist in the third interspace [5], but is clinically seen commonly in the second interspace [50]. In the author's opinion, the presence of either a first or fourth interspace forefoot nerve entrapment is extremely rare. In more than a decade of performing endoscopic decompression of forefoot nerve entrapments, the author has only released one fourth interspace, with improvement noted by the patient.

The specific surgical indication for EDIN-2 (endoscopic decompression of intermetatarsal nerve—second generation) is for primary release of forefoot interspace nerve entrapment. The procedure is not indicated for intervention where there exists a recurrent Morton's neuroma. However, the author has had reports from several surgeons who have had success with endoscopic decompression of previously operated interspaces, in addition to successful performance of decompression on five previously operated interspaces. It is hypothesized that nothing more than a release of fibrotic tissue occurs from the endoscopic decompression. In these anecdotal cases, improvement and in most cases complete resolution has been seen, but to explain the physiological basis is difficult. It may be nothing more than a release of the scar tissue in the interspace, which somehow alleviates pressure on the end bulb neuroma, thereby eliminating the patient's discomfort.

EDIN-2

Either general or local anesthesia with monitored sedation can be used for this surgical technique. Once trained, after overcoming the learning curve, the technique rarely takes more than 10 minutes. The anesthesia team can lend assistance in determining what type of sedation they would like to use based on the length of the procedure. While straight local anesthesia is an acceptable method for this procedure, one must not infiltrate anesthesia into the operative site. In contrast to arthroscopies, where a fluid environment is ideal, this operative area must be kept dry. Any local anesthesia that leaks into the cannula will only obscure the surgeon's view, making the procedure difficult.

The patient should be placed on the operating room table in a supine position. The patient's feet should not hang off the operating room table (this is opposite of the first generation EDIN technique). Use of an ankle tourniquet is optimal, and should be well padded. Standard intraoperative preparation is used for a sterile set-up. Hemostasis is imperative to the success of any endoscopic surgical technique. The foot should be exsanguinated with an Esmark bandage, followed by inflation of an ankle tourniquet to 250 mm Hg. Exsanguination with an ACE-type elastic bandage is not ideal. Topographical markings with a skin scribe will aid the surgeon in instrument placement, as well as ensuring that no vital structures are mistakenly severed (see Fig. 4).

The essential goal of the EDIN-2 surgical technique is to atraumatically insert the oval cannula/obturator under the transverse metatarsal ligament from the digital webspace. This will place the plantar neurovascular structures beneath the cannula, protecting them, while at the same time allow for maximal visualization of the plantar aspect of the transverse intermetatarsal ligament (TIML). As can be seen in Fig. 5, proper placement of the instrumentation has occurred, which allows the visualization that is seen in Fig. 6.

Once complete transection of the TIML is seen endoscopically, the instrumentation is removed, and the elevator is placed into the webspace incision to tactilely verify that there are no fibers of the TIML remaining. The surgeon will be able to easily move this instrument up and down between the respective metatarsal heads without any resistance. This assures the surgeon that the area is adequately decompressed.

EDIN-2 surgical technique summary

1. Patient is in a supine position with an ankle tourniquet inflated to 250 mm Hg.
2. Local anesthesia with IV monitored anesthesia care, consisting of a posterior tibial block and anterior ankle block. **All attention is directed to avoiding infiltration of any anesthetic into the interspace area.**
3. Palpate from dorsal to plantar between the metatarsal heads of the affected interspace, and then use a skin scribe to mark a transverse line about 2 to 2.5 cm proximal from the level of the metatarsalphalangeal joints.
4. A similar mark will be made in the affected webspace, in a transverse manner located at the midpoint of the web from dorsal to plantar, to be between the dorsal and plantar neurovascular bundles.
5. A linear line is drawn on the dorsal aspect of the foot to correspond to the angle of the diaphysis of the metatarsals. This will be used by the

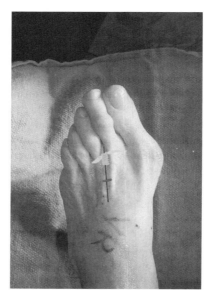

Fig. 4. This illustrates demarcation of the topographic anatomy to ensure proper incision placement and avoidance of the long flexor tendon.

surgeon when placing the instrumentation so that a flexor tendon is not
crossed.

6. The foot is exsanguinated with an Esmark bandage and the ankle cuff
is inflated.

7. The dorsal incision is made, about 5 to 6 mm in a transverse manner, at
the marked level as indicated in step 3, and the surgeon is careful to
ensure that the blade is not deeper than just below the dermis to avoid
transection of any superficial peroneal nerve branches.

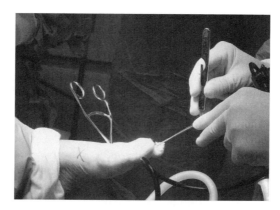

Fig. 5. Proper orientation of the EDIN-2 instrumentation.

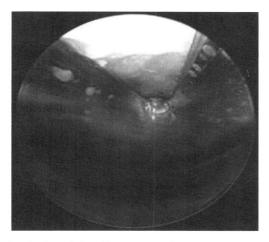

Fig. 6. Illustrates visualization of the white transverse intermetatarsal ligament before cutting.

8. Steven's tenotomy scissors are then placed into the incision, that allows spreading of the subcutaneous tissue, and this will allow placement of the metatarsal spreader between the metatarsal shafts. The scissors should be placed deep enough so that when they are spread, the surgeon will be able to feel the metatarsals.

9. A similar incision as described in step 7 is made, transversely, measuring up to a centimeter. Careful attention is made not to bury the blade so that the small nerves are not transected.

10. Blunt dissection is made from a dorsal distal to plantar proximal direction so that the distal aspect of the TIML is able to be palpated with the elevator. Attention should be paid to this step, as it is necessary to be aggressive enough so that there are no subcutaneous fibers, which will impair placement of the cannula, but at the same time the surgeon should be very careful not to disrupt tissue unnecessarily. **Remember: the TIML is at the plantar aspect of the metatarsal heads.**

11. The surgeon will now palpate the TIML, on its inferior surface, and then drop the hand so as to direct the elevator proximally in essentially the same angle as the metatarsal inclination angle. This only takes two-finger pencil grip strength to achieve, and if more resistance is met, then the surgeon should be aware that they are not in the correct tissue plane, and therefore redirect their instrumentation. Once this step has been achieved, the surgeon should then try to feel the resistance of the TIML with trying to move the elevator superiorly. This is important so that there is a psychomotor reference after the surgeon completes the transection of the TIML, and can distinguish the difference of resistance. There will be no resistance with dorsal elevation of the instrument when the TIML has been adequately transected. The

surgeon should feel the instrument "pop" up and down between the
met heads.

12. The obturator/cannula should then be placed into the foot in an identical manner as just described. The cannula should be placed so that
the hub is about the level of the distal interphalangeal joints, and
should not be buried all the way into the webspace.

13. The obturator is removed, and can be swabbed out if necessary with
a cotton-tipped applicator.

14. The scope (2.7-mm 30-degree bevel, min 150 mm in length) should then
be gripped with the surgeon's nondominant hand, and placed into the
side of the oval cannula with the bevel angled toward the midline of the
slot, and the TIML can then be visualized. The proximal and distal
margins of the TIML should be identified, and then the surgeon should
move the scope to visualize the proximal margin, and hold the scope
there.

15. The surgeon will then introduce the angled hook knife into the other
side of the oval cannula, and this will allow for visualization of the
hook when the blade is introduced to the level of the proximal margin
of the TIML.

16. The blade should be engaged into the proximal margin of the TIML,
and then both the scope and the blade withdrawn from the cannula.
This will allow visualization of the cut being made.

17. Several passes with the hook knife may be necessary to adequately release the ligament.

18. Once the surgeon feels that the TIML has been adequately transected,
then the metatarsal retractor can be retracted more, and the severed
edges of the TIML can be visualized as separating.

19. The obturator is reintroduced into the cannula, and both are then
withdrawn.

20. The elevator is then replaced into the interspace, and the surgeon
should be able to pass the instrument dorsally and plantarly between
the metatarsal heads without resistance. If the elevator is placed far
enough into the foot, there will always be resistance because the instrument will be proximal to the tissue that has been decompressed. The
surgeon can place the finger on the elevator at the webspace, and
then withdraw the instrument and then place it on the dorsal aspect
of the foot to see how far proximal it is that tissue is being felt.

21. Skin closure is achieved with simple interrupted 5-0 sutures.

22. A small compressive gauze dressing is then placed on the foot.

Postoperative management

Because the EDIN-2 is minimally traumatic, patients are allowed to remove their own dressing the next morning after surgery. They are instructed
that they may shower regularly, but they are not to immerse their foot in

water like a hot tub or a swimming pool. They can return to a regular shoe, which is comfortable and does not cause them any discomfort, or they can continue with their surgical shoe. Sutures are removed 10 to 14 days after surgery. They may perform any activity that does not cause them pain, or swelling. Usually, they can begin to return to athletics between the fourth and sixth week. By the eighth week, they usually have no restrictions to activity. Occasionally, if they have some neuritis after the third week, they may be given a steroid injection. Patients are instructed preoperatively that their final result will not be determined until 16 weeks postdecompression. If a patient is not improved at 16 weeks, it is very likely that he or she will not have an ideal surgical result, and may need additional intervention.

Complications

Postoperative complications with the EDIN-2 technique are rare. While there has been a report of transection of the plantar plate and flexor digitorum longus tendon [51], overall complications with the technique have been minimal, rare, and when they do occur, they usually consist of minor skin infections of the portal incisions. There have been a few isolated reports of formation of hammer digit syndrome following endoscopic decompression of the intermetatarsal space, but in all cases reviewed by the author, there had been a series of local anesthetic steroid injections given in the affected interspace before surgical intervention. It is a well-known complication of steroid injections given in the intermetatarsal space for the development of plantar plate rupture with resulting pre-dislocation syndrome, with contracture and medial or lateral deviation at the level of the metatarsal phalangeal joint. This is seen often in patients who never had any type of surgery. Conjecture about the impairment of lumbricle tendon function as a possible etiology for this development post–endoscopic decompression exists. This biomechanical theory is likely erroneous for two reasons. First, there are a significant number of humans who don't have lumbricle tendons anatomically to begin with. Secondly, the lumbricle tendon uses the transverse intermetatarsal ligament as a fulcrum, and even if the tendon itself was not transected, in nearly every surgical procedure, open or endoscopic, the treatment of Morton's entrapment involves cutting of this ligament, which effectively renders this tendon to a nonfunctional state. Development of hammer digit syndrome has not occurred in even a small percentage of these procedures—far from it, as it is a truly rare complication. It is disruption of the plantar plate that is the more likely contributor toward development of contracture at the level of the metatarsalphalangeal joint, and the surgeon should caution those patients who have had prior steroid, alcohol injections, or cryoablation procedures that they may be at more risk for development of hammer digit syndrome after any type of interspace surgery that involves transection of the TIML.

Finally, it is fair to say that the risks and complications associated with decompression, endoscopic or open, of forefoot nerve entrapments are far less and serious than those seen with resection or destruction of the nerve. There are numerous patients whose lives have been destroyed by the "simple Morton's neuroma" resection, who are living in and out of tertiary pain clinics because of formation of a true amputation neuroma. There has never been a report of development of an amputation neuroma post–endoscopic decompression.

Surgical results

Results of 69 patients, accounting for 96 interspaces were recently reported in a retrospective review from 1993 to 1999, with an overall success rate of excellent/good results in 75 interspaces (86.2%) [52]. Twelve interspaces were categorized as poor (13.7%). It should be noted that some of the interspaces that were ultimately classified as poor had prior treatment with sclerosing injections, which had previously damaged the peripheral nerve. In the future, selection criteria for patients to be decompressed may not include those with previous attempts of destructive procedures like cryoablation and alcohol sclerosing injections. We also noted a decrease in overall success rate when adjacent interspace decompressions were performed. In fact, when those patients who had prior nerve destructive procedures, and or adjacent interspace involvement, were removed from the study, there was an overall success rate of 91.3%.

This compares very favorably with not only reports of Morton's resection, but also with results reported with open neurolysis by Dellon [53], Guathier [54], and Vito and Talarico [55]. Recently, Shapiro [56] reported excellent preliminary results in 40 patients with a different endoscopic system. As of this time, there have been no published results from blind techniques of neurolysis.

Summary

Our experience since 1992 with endoscopic decompression for forefoot nerve entrapments, in addition to the published data, support further implementation of this lesser invasive surgical technique for the treatment of Morton's entrapment. With improvements in diagnostic technology, such as musculoskeletal ultrasound and neurosensory testing, in addition to enhanced clinical recognition of coexistent pathology such as tarsal tunnel syndrome and equinus, the modern day foot and ankle specialist is far ahead of where the specialist was just one decade ago. Also, the slow professional recognition of "Morton's Neuroma" as a true nerve entrapment phenomenon, leading toward decompression/neurolysis, will only continue to improve patient outcomes.

References

[1] Kinley S, Frascone S, Calderone D, et al. Endoscopic plantar fasciotomy versus traditional heel spur surgery: a prospective study. J Foot Ankle Surg 1993;32(6):595–603.

[2] Tomczak RL, Haverstock BD. A retrospective comparison of endoscopic plantar fasciotomy to open plantar fasciotomy with heel spur resection for chronic plantar fasciitis/heel spur syndrome. J Foot Ankle Surg 1995;34(3):305–11.

[3] Hoadley AE. Six Cases of metatarsalgia. The Chicago Medical Reporter 1893;5:32–7.

[4] Levy M, Seelenfreund M, Maor P, et al. [Post-traumatic Morton's neuroma] Harefuah 1972;83(5):202–3.

[5] Larson EE, Barrett SL, Battison B, et al. Accurate nomenclature of forefoot nerve entrapment: a historical perspective. J Am Podiatr Med Assoc 2005;95(3):298–306.

[6] Bruner JM. Carpal tunnel syndrome. Hand 1972;4(3):220–3.

[7] Civinini F. Su di un ganglare rigonflamento della pinata del plede. Mem Chir Archiespedale Pistola;1835. p. 4–17.

[8] Morton TG. A peculiar and painful affection of the fourth metatarsalphalangeal articulation. Am J Med Sci 1876;71:37–45.

[9] Durlacher LA. Treatise on corns, bunions, the diseases of nails, and the general management of the feet;1845. p. 52.

[10] Vogel FCW. Klinik der Gelenkkrankheiten. 1st edition. 1877. p. 339–51.

[11] Morton TSK. Metatarsalgia (Morton's painful affection of the foot) with an account of six cases cured by operation. 1893.

[12] MacKinnon SE, Dellon AL. Surgery of the peripheral nerve. 1988.

[13] Morscher E, Ulrich J, Dick W. Morton's intermetatarsal neuroma: morphology and histological substrate. Foot Ankle Int 2000;21(7):558–62.

[14] Graham CE, Graham DM. Morton's neuroma: A microscopic evaluation. Foot and Ankle 1984;5:150–3.

[15] Shereff M, Grande DA. Electron microscopy of the interdigital neuroma. Clin Orthop 1991; 271:296–9.

[16] Caporusso EF, Fallat LM, Savoy-Moore R. Cryogenic neuroablation for the treatment of lower extremity neuromas. J Foot Ankle Surg 2002;41(5):286–90.

[17] Dockery GL. The treatment of intermetatarsal neuromas with 4% alcohol sclerosing injections. J Foot Ankle Surg 1999;38(6):403–8.

[18] Finney W, Wiener SN, Catanzariti F. Treatment of Morton's neuroma using percutaneous electrocoagulation. J Am Podiatr Med Assoc 1989;79(12):615–8.

[19] Smith HP, McWhorter JM, Challa VR. Radiofrequency neurolysis in a clinical model. Neuropathological correlation. J Neurosurg 1981;55(2):246–53.

[20] Sunderland S. The restoration of median nerve function after destructive lesions which preclude end-to-end repair. Brain 1974;97(1):1–14.

[21] Sunderland S. The anatomic foundation of peripheral nerve repair techniques. Orthop Clin North Am 1981;12(2):245–66.

[22] Sunderland S. The anatomy and physiology of nerve injury. Muscle Nerve 1990;13(9): 771–84.

[23] Dellon AL. Somatosensory testing and rehabilitation. 2000.

[24] Schneider RK, Mayhew IG, Clarke GL. Effects of cryotherapy on the palmar and plantar digital nerves in the horse. Am J Vet Res 1985;46(1):7–12.

[25] Davies E, Pounder D, Mansour S, et al. Cryosurgery for chronic injuries of the cutaneous nerve in the upper limb. Analysis of a new open technique. J Bone Joint Surg Br 2000; 82(3):413–5.

[26] Youngswick FD. Intermetatarsal neuroma. Clin Podiatr Med Surg 1994;11(4):579–92.

[27] Mulder JD. The causative mechanism in Morton's metatarsalgia. J Bone Joint Surg Br 1951; 33-B(1):94–5.

[28] Beggs I. Sonographic appearances of nerve tumors. J Clin Ultrasound 1999;27(7):363–8.

[29] Ernberg LA, Adler RS, Lane J. Ultrasound in the detection and treatment of a painful stump neuroma. Skeletal Radiol 2003;32(5):306–9.
[30] Kaminsky S, Griffin L, Milsap J, et al. Is ultrasonography a reliable way to confirm the diagnosis of Morton's neuroma? Orthopedics 1997;20(1):37–9.
[31] Oliver TB, Beggs I. Ultrasound in the assessment of metatarsalgia: a surgical and histological correlation. Clin Radiol 1998;53(4):287–9.
[32] Peer S, Kovacs P, Harff C, et al. High-resolution sonography of lower extremity peripheral nerves: anatomic correlation and spectrum of disease. J Ultrasound Med 2002;21(3):315–22.
[33] Pollak RA, Bellacosa RA, Dornbluth NC, et al. Sonographic analysis of Morton's neuroma. J Foot Surg 1992;31(6):534–7.
[34] Quinn TJ, Jacobson JA, Craig JG, et al. Sonography of Morton's neuromas. AJR Am J Roentgenol 2000;174(6):1723–8.
[35] Shapiro PP, Shapiro SL. Sonographic evaluation of interdigital neuromas. Foot Ankle Int 1995;16(10):604–6.
[36] Sobiesk GA, Wertheimer SJ, Schulz R, et al. Sonographic evaluation of interdigital neuromas. J Foot Ankle Surg 1997;36(5):364–6.
[37] Baert AL, Sartor K. High resolution sonography of the peripheral nervous system. 2003.
[38] Timins ME. MR imaging of the foot and ankle. Foot Ankle Clin 2000;5(1):83–101 [vi.].
[39] Williams JW, Meaney J, Whitehouse GH, et al. MRI in the investigation of Morton's neuroma: which sequences? Clin Radiol 1997;52(1):46–9.
[40] Zanetti M, Ledermann T, Zollinger H, et al. Efficacy of MR imaging in patients suspected of having Morton's neuroma. AJR Am J Roentgenol 1997;168(2):529–32.
[41] Younger AS, Claridge RJ. The role of diagnostic block in the management of Morton's neuroma. Can J Surg 1998;41(2):127–30.
[42] Hogan QH, Abram SE. Neural blockade for diagnosis and prognosis. A review. Anesthesiology 1997;86(1):216–41.
[43] Dellon AL. Treatment of recurrent metatarsalgia by neuroma resection and muscle implantation: case report and proposed algorithm of management for Morton's "neuroma." Microsurgery 1989;10(3):256–9.
[44] Jacoby R. Neuroma pain as a metabolic marker. Presented at the IPNS 2004 Annual Meeting. Las Vegas, NV. October 3–5, 2005.
[45] Lavery LA, Armstrong DG, Boulton AJ. Ankle equinus deformity and its relationship to high plantar pressure in a large population with diabetes mellitus. J Am Podiatr Med Assoc 2002;92(9):479–82.
[46] Lin SS, Lee TH, Wapner KL. Plantar forefoot ulceration with equinus deformity of the ankle in diabetic patients: the effect of tendo-Achilles lengthening and total contact casting. Orthopedics 1996;19(5):465–75.
[47] McGlamry ED, Butlin WE, Ruch JA. Treatment of forefoot equinus by tendon transpositions. J Am Podiatry Assoc 1975;65(9):872–88.
[48] Subotnick SI. Equinus deformity as it affects the forefoot. J Am Podiatry Assoc 1971;61(11):423–7.
[49] Barrett SL, Jarvis J. Consideration of equinus in forefoot nerve entrapments–treatment via endoscopic gastrocnemius recession (EGR): a clinical case example. Submitted to J Am Podiatr Med Assoc 2005;95(5):464–8.
[50] Keh RA, Ballew KK, Higgins KR, et al. Long-term follow-up of Morton's neuroma. J Foot Surg 1992;31(1):93–5.
[51] Brodsky JW, Passmore RN, Shabat S. Transection of the plantar plate and the flexor digitorum longus tendon of the fourth toe as a complication of endoscopic treatment of interdigiatal neuroma: a case report. J Bone Joint Surg 2004;86-A(Number 10): 2299–301.
[52] Barrett SL, Walsh A. A retrospective study of endoscopic decompression of intermetatarsal nerve entrapment (EDIN). J Am Podiatr Med Assoc 2006;96(1):19–29.

[53] Dellon AL. Treatment of Morton's neuroma as a nerve compression. The role for neurolysis. J Am Podiatr Med Assoc 1992;82(8):399–402.
[54] Gauthier G. Thomas Morton's disease: a nerve entrapment syndrome. A new surgical technique. Clin Orthop 1979;142:90–2.
[55] Vito GR, Talarico LM. A modified technique for Morton's neuroma. Decompression with relocation. J Am Podiatr Med Assoc 2003;93(3):190–4.
[56] Shapiro SL. Endoscopic decompression of the intermetatarsal nerve for Morton's neuroma. Foot Ankle Clin 2004;9(2):297–304.

ELSEVIER
SAUNDERS

Clin Podiatr Med Surg
23 (2006) 597–609

CLINICS IN
PODIATRIC
MEDICINE AND
SURGERY

Tarsal Tunnel Syndrome: A Compression Neuropathy Involving Four Distinct Tunnels

Justin Franson, DPM[a], Babak Baravarian, DPM[b],*

[a]Foot and Ankle Institute of Valencia, 26357 MC Bean Parkway, Suite 250,
Valencia, CA 91355, USA
[b]Foot and Ankle Institute of Santa Monica, 2121 Wilshire Boulevard, Suite 101,
Santa Monica, CA 90403, USA

Tarsal tunnel syndrome is a more common condition of the foot and ankle than has been historically appreciated in the literature. In 1933, Pollock and Davis [1] referred to a compression of the posterior tibial nerve secondary to traumatic fibrosis. In 1960, Koppel [2] described the symptoms of tarsal tunnel syndrome. Later, it earned the name "tarsal tunnel syndrome" when Keck [3] and Lam [4] independently published articles in 1962. Currently, it is a condition that is largely under-diagnosed as a potential cause of heel pain, arch pain, and distal peripheral neuropathy. Because the symptoms can mirror those associated with other lower extremity conditions, it can easily be missed by the practitioner, even the lower extremity specialist [5]. False-negative electrodiagnostic testing contributes to the under-diagnosis of tarsal tunnel syndrome, the most common chronic nerve entrapment in the lower extremity [6].

Tarsal tunnel syndrome is a peripheral compression neuropathy of the tibial nerve and its branches, which results in a range of neuritic symptoms that affect the plantar aspect of the foot. Compression of the branches of the tibial nerve has been referred to as "distal tarsal tunnel syndrome" [7]. Patients often complain of sensory disturbances to portions of the foot, localized or radiating pain, burning pain, paresthesias, disturbances in the perception of temperature (feelings of coldness), or feeling as though there is a tight band around the foot. However, in certain cases, there is no associated tingling and only a mild sensory loss or irritation of the pad and sole of the foot or heel is noted. Pain is often felt later in the development of chronic

* Corresponding author.
   E-mail address: bbaravarian@mednet.ucla.edu (B. Baravarian).

0891-8422/06/$ - see front matter © 2006 Elsevier Inc. All rights reserved.
doi:10.1016/j.cpm.2006.04.005   *podiatric.theclinics.com*

tarsal tunnel syndrome, and is a less common complaint [6]. Although distal radiation of symptoms is the norm, proximal radiation of symptoms can and does occur in some cases of tarsal tunnel syndrome. Distal lower extremity symptoms are often attributed to a more proximal etiology, such as sciatica or radiculopathy. In a similar manner, distal compression neuropathy can cause more proximal symptoms.

Tarsal tunnel syndrome has historically been compared with, and even said to be analogous to, the well-known carpal tunnel syndrome [7,5,8]. However, it has been more recently distinguished from carpal tunnel syndrome, because of differences in anatomy, etiology, treatment, and response to treatment [6,9]. The tarsal tunnel is more analogous to the distal portion of the forearm rather than the carpal tunnel. Although synovium is present in the carpal tunnel, it is not present in the tarsal tunnel [6].

Anatomy

Tibial nerve

The sciatic nerve is formed from spinal cord segments L4 to S2; as it proceeds in the lower extremity, it branches at the popliteal fossa into the tibial nerve and the common peroneal nerve. The tibial nerve, the larger of the two branches, passes between the two heads of the gastrocnemius muscle to the medial aspect of the ankle.

As the tibial nerve passes into the tarsal tunnel, the distal branching pattern has been shown to be variable. In most cadaver specimens studied (93%–95%) [6], the medial and lateral plantar nerves have been shown to bifurcate while still in the anatomic tarsal tunnel [10,11]. In a smaller percentage of feet, 5%–7%, the bifurcation occurs above, or proximal to, the entrance to the tarsal tunnel. Dellon [10] theorized that this may predispose these patients to develop tarsal tunnel because of a larger cross-sectional area of the nerves as they pass into the tight anatomic space entering the tarsal tunnel.

The medial calcaneal nerve usually branches from the tibial nerve, although it has also been shown to branch from the lateral plantar nerve less commonly [9–11], 25% of the time, according to one source [11]. Havel and colleagues [11] showed the medial calcaneal nerve to have multiple branches off the tibial nerve 21% of the time. The medial calcaneal nerve pierces the flexor retinaculum, or will pass inferior to it, providing sensory innervation to the posterior and medial aspects of the heel.

The medial and lateral plantar nerves supply autonomic, sensory, and motor fibers to the plantar foot [12]. These two nerve branches exit the tarsal tunnel, course through about 1 cm of fatty tissue, and then enter into their own tunnels. As they pass the fascial origin of the abductor hallucis, the nerves are divided by a firm septum that attaches to the calcaneus or the flexor tendon sheaths [10]. The medial plantar nerve passes deep to the abductor hallucis and flexor hallucis longus muscles, and then divides into three common digital nerves. The lateral plantar nerve passes directly through the abductor hallucis muscle belly as it passes to the lateral foot before its terminal division.

Peripheral nerves are enclosed in three layers of tissue. The innermost layer, the endoneurium, contains the functional nerve fibers. This is surrounded by the perineurium, a thin but strong layer of connective tissue which protects the underlying nerve fibers. The nerve is further embedded in the epineurium, a loose connective tissue layer.

Tarsal tunnel

The tarsal tunnel is an area of anatomic narrowing caused by tight ligamentous structures. It is a fibro-osseous tunnel bordered superficially by the flexor retinaculum (or laciniate ligament), which passes obliquely from posterior to anterior. The flexor retinaculum forms the roof of the tarsal tunnel, as well as the superior and inferior margins. The floor of the tunnel is formed by the medial wall of the talus and calcaneus and the distal medial wall of the tibia.

The anatomic structures that course within the tarsal tunnel are, from medial to lateral, the posterior tibial tendon, flexor digitorum longus tendon, posterior tibial artery and its accompanying veins, posterior tibial nerve, and the flexor hallucis longus tendon.

Etiology

What causes tarsal tunnel syndrome? It is a compression neuropathy of the posterior tibial nerve as it passes in the anatomic tarsal tunnel in the medial ankle under flexor retinaculum. In a literature review of tarsal tunnel syndrome, it was estimated that in 60%–80% of cases, the specific cause can be identified [9].

Tarsal tunnel syndrome can be attributed to causes that lie within the anatomic confines of the tarsal tunnel, often caused by "space-occupying lesions," or from forces or factors external to the tarsal tunnel. Some etiologic entities include osseous prominences (post-traumatic or otherwise), trauma, generalized lower extremity edema, heel varus or valgus or the compensation for these hindfoot deformities, soft tissue masses such as ganglia or lipoma, neurilemoma, varicosities or venous congestion, tendon pathology, post-traumatic peri-neural fibrosis, systemic inflammatory arthridities, diabetes, hypertrophic flexor retinaculum, post-surgical scarring, and an anomalous muscle [13,14].

Abnormal pronation and its relationship to the development of tarsal tunnel syndrome has been disputed in the literature [15]. Although it may contribute to the development or worsening of many foot conditions, the debate focuses on whether it is a pure etiologic factor in the development of tarsal tunnel syndrome [15,16]. An entrapment of the first branch of the lateral plantar nerve, termed "Baxter's nerve," is exacerbated not by a pronated foot type, but by supinatory positions.

It has been suggested that chronic intractable heel pain is often caused by entrapment neuropathy. One article presented 51 patients in a study of chronic heel pain syndrome, all of whom had entrapment neuropathy [17].

Peripheral nerves are rendered more sensitive or susceptible to damage if there is a more proximal nerve lesion or pathology. Tarsal tunnel syndrome can be triggered as sequelae of proximal nerve damage; this idea has been referred to as the "double-crush" phenomenon. As reported by Persich [8], this hypothesis, which originated from Upton and McComas, is that local damage to a nerve at a proximal level makes that nerve more susceptible to damage distal to the lesion.

Diagnosis

The diagnosis of tarsal tunnel syndrome is based largely upon the patient history combined with clinical exam; adjunctive imaging and diagnostic testing can provide additional supporting information to strengthen or confirm the clinical diagnosis. Patients will usually present with some level of neuritic symptoms, including sensory disturbances such as tingling, numbness, burning, or pain. These sensations can be observed at the toes, metatarsal level, through the arch, or at the heel; there may be occasional proximal radiation of symptoms. The condition will typically worsen as a result of certain activities, including prolonged standing or walking. Night symptoms are not uncommon, especially after a day of extended weight-bearing activity. Rest and leg elevation will often relieve symptoms. Tarsal tunnel syndrome does not include symptoms that affect the dorsal or lateral aspect of the foot.

Clinical examination may or may not reveal significant findings. A positive Tinel's sign upon percussion of the tibial nerve is a strong positive indicator of tarsal tunnel syndrome and is often present. Pain and deep palpation along the posterior tibial nerve is also consistent with tarsal tunnel syndrome. Swelling in the tarsal tunnel and into the medial arch is sometimes present, which suggests the possible presence of a space-occupying lesion.

Weakness of the intrinsics can occur as tarsal tunnel syndrome progresses and in chronic, long-standing cases. Secondary toe contractures can be a long-term result of tarsal tunnel syndrome.

Clinical maneuvers designed to increase the pressure on the posterior tibial nerve in the tarsal tunnel have been described in the literature over the years [18]. A modification to the classic dorsiflexion-eversion test was presented in 2001, as a diagnostic indicator of tarsal tunnel syndrome. The test is performed by placing the ankle in maximum eversion and dorsiflexion, while maximally dorsiflexing the toes at the metatarsophalan-geal joints. This position is held for 5–10 seconds; exacerbation of symptoms is thought to be diagnostic [19].

Diagnostic studies

If a physician is suspicious of a systemic arthritis or other inflammatory processes, laboratory studies should be ordered. Screening for systemic conditions such as diabetes or thyroid dysfunction can be ordered when appropriate [7].

Imaging studies can include foot and ankle radiographs, followed by computed tomography (CT) when appropriate to further evaluate any osseous prominences, coalition, or other structural abnormality. Lumbar spine radiographs and MRI can be included as part of a complete work-up of a peripheral nerve condition, or if the physician suspects a proximal nerve etiology that may be contributing to a "double-crush" phenomenon.

MRI can be ordered especially if there is clinical evidence of a space-occupying lesion. Some studies have reported MRI to be highly accurate (82%–83%) in the diagnosis of tarsal tunnel syndrome [12].

Diagnostic ultrasound can be used to check for synovitis of peripheral tendon sheaths such as the posterior tibial and flexor tendons about the ankle. Ganglia and space- occupying lesions can also be identified in the region of the tarsal tunnel or surrounding structures. The tibial nerve and its branches can also be traced to evaluate the potential presence of a high division; this can result in overfill of the tarsal canal by the medial and lateral plantar nerve branches. Tests are often performed using a high-frequency type machine and a 10–15 mhz linear probe.

When suspicious of a pathologic venous network in the tarsal tunnel, it may be useful to stimulating venous engorgement with the use of a tourniquet proximal to the tarsal tunnel [12]. Exacerbation or re-creation of symptoms with this test can help identify the specific etiology of the tarsal tunnel syndrome.

Electrodiagnostic studies have traditionally been the gold standard for confirming and evaluating the clinical diagnosis of tarsal tunnel syndrome. Motor and sensory nerve conduction studies (NCS) and electromyography (EMG) should be evaluated. EMG may show motor latencies in the abductor hallucis or abductor digiti minimi. It has been suggested that sensory action potentials is a more sensitive test. False negative NCS and EMG are not uncommon, and so unfortunately, do not rule out tarsal tunnel syndrome.

A more recent diagnostic tool is computer-assisted quantitative sensory testing, also known as a pressure-specified sensory device or PSSD [6]. This neurosensory testing device has been shown to provide a more sensitive appreciation of peripheral nerve compromise, which can confirm a clinical diagnosis earlier in the progression of tarsal tunnel syndrome. Studies have shown that prolonged nerve compression leads to a lower rate of positive surgical outcomes [14]. The PSSD machine is designed to address the subtle changes that occur in peripheral nerves as nerve damage increases. One- and two-point static discrimination are used in pre-operative testing and moving one- and two-point discrimination are used in early post-operative testing. An article by Soomekh and colleagues in this clinics issue is devoted to the development and philosophy behind the PSSD device.

Treatment

To increase the rate of positive outcomes, management of tarsal tunnel syndrome should be directed at the specific etiologic agent. As mentioned above, in 60%–80% of cases of tarsal tunnel syndrome, the specific cause can be identified [9].

Conservative treatment

Conservative management of tarsal tunnel syndrome can include taping, bracing, stretching, icing, or the use of orthotics, shoe modifications, massage, ultrasound, and aspiration of ganglia. As is true for many conditions of the foot and ankle, surgical intervention is pursued after a failed course of conservative treatment. Studies have reported that prolonged tarsal tunnel syndrome has a lower rate of positive surgical outcomes [14]. Based upon this, the authors recommend that surgical intervention be considered if conservative measures do not provide benefit in the short term. The threshold for failed conservative treatment may need to be lowered; an arbitrarily time period for failing conservative methods cannot be justified. Although it is difficult to define a specific threshold for abandoning conservative care, it is important to remember that the longer a patient has tarsal tunnel syndrome, the greater the potential for lasting nerve damage.

Surgical treatment

A diagnosis of tarsal tunnel syndrome should be confirmed by NCS, EMG, or PSSD tests before surgical intervention. A positive Tinel's sign seems to be an indicator of this condition; when present, there is a higher likelihood that the patient will do well after surgery. If there are sensory deficits in the absence of a positive Tinel's sign, surgery may have a lower chance of recovering the nerve function [6].

The authors believe that certain instruments can be used to optimize the performance of the surgical procedure. These include a blunt-tip iris scissor, a small and large army/navy retractor, and an Adson-type bipolar cautery. Furthermore, to perform an internal neurolysis of the nerve, in addition to loupe magnification, microscopic curved and straight scissors as well as atraumatic forceps are recommended. The authors prefer to perform the procedure under loop magnification ×6, but the use of loop magnification ×2 or ×3 or a microscope for the internal neurolysis may also be sufficient.

An open surgical approach is preferred by the authors who use a thigh pneumatic tourniquet. The incision is centered between the medial malleolus and the posterior Achilles tendon region (Fig. 1). It is important to avoid placing the incision too close to the medial malleolus, because this introduces a greater possibility of damage to the posterior branch of the saphenous nerve. The incision is extended distally over the abductor hallucis muscle belly region with a linear or a slight curve anteriorly as needed to place the distal incision over the muscle belly just proximal to its calcaneal insertion.

When the skin incision has been made, dissection is deepened with blunt technique to avoid inadvertent laceration of nerve branches, which could compromise an otherwise successful tarsal tunnel release by the formation of a painful nerve ending. Blunt dissection is performed in a linear fashion to the level of the flexor retinaculum. The small perforating vessels are cauterized as necessary with the use of the Adson bipolar forceps; which minimizes the potential thermal damage to the adjacent soft tissues.

When the flexor retinaculum is identified, this tight fascial layer is lifted and a small stab incision is made into the central portion. A blunt device can then be introduced under the retinaculum to protect the nerve. It is not uncommon to find that the tibial nerve retinaculum is not very tight and the main region of compression is farther distal (Fig. 2). The retinaculum is released along its entire course from the level of the dorsal abductor

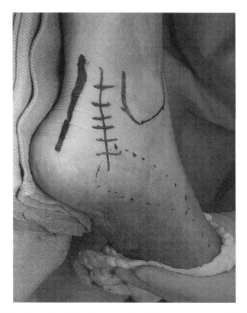

Fig. 1. Tarsal tunnel incision. Incision is centralized between the Achilles tendon and medial malleolus and extends over the adductor muscle belly.

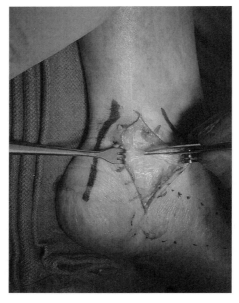

Fig. 2. Tarsal tunnel laxity. The actual tarsal tunnel region is lax compared with the tightness of the adductor muscle belly tunnel regions.

muscle belly to the proximal border. When the release is complete, the contents of the tarsal tunnel can be visualized. The tibial nerve and any perforating or calcaneal branches are identified (Fig. 3). Extensive dissection should be avoided. A space-occupying lesion, when present, should be dissected free and excised en toto. The venous structures should be examined for tortuous or irregular anatomy and ligated as necessary if pathologic.

The superficial fascia that overlays the abductor muscle belly is identified and released (Fig. 4). The muscle belly is then carefully retracted plantarly using an army/navy retractor and the deep fascia of the abductor muscle belly is identified. This is the region of greatest compression in most cases and the region that is most often not addressed during tarsal tunnel release (which likely results in a percentage of the failed releases). Two distinct tunnels are identified that divide the medial and lateral plantar nerves in the region of the deep abductor retinaculum (Fig. 5). A straight hemostat is passed gently along the tunnel site to check for tightness. When the tunnel is identified, care is taken to protect the nerve and venous plexus and a blunt-tip iris scissor is used to release the tunnel along its course. Both tunnels are fully released and then the central fibrous septa, which divides the two tunnels, is resected to make one large passage for both nerves. It is important to remove the central septa to prevent fibrosis and to enlarge the entrance of the nerves into the foot. The calcaneal nerves are also identified and the tunnels that run to the heel region are released along the medial

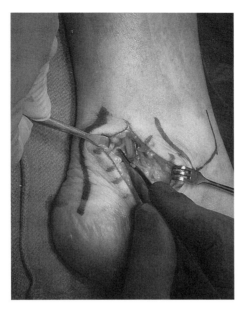

Fig. 3. Calcaneal nerve branch. The calcaneal nerve branch extends off the tibial nerve region.

heel region. There is a distinct tunnel for each calcaneal nerve branch as it passes below the abductor retinaculum into the plantar heel region. Each branch identified (usually one or two) is freed into the heel area when the overlying superficial retinaculum is released.

A bipolar device is used to cauterize the edges of the retinaculum to allow shrinkage of the tissue and prevent the possibility of reattachment. Any small vessels noted are also cauterized; care must be taken to protect the nerve branches.

The tibial nerve and the medial and lateral plantar nerves are then checked for internal fibrosis. The goal is to be able to see the distinct fascicles of nerve without fibrosis. This is best evaluated under loop magnification. If fibrosis is noted, microscopic instrumentation is used to make a linear incision into the perineurium and free the fascicle branches. There is no need to spread the perineurium; the essential factor in this part of the surgery is to free the circumferential fibrosis with a linear release. The most common region of fibrosis is the distal tibial nerve at its division point; there is not much need for treatment of the medial or lateral plantar branches because they are not often found to have heavy fibrosis.

The wound is closed with simple buried absorbable suture at the subcutaneous level and skin closure with either nylon suture or staples. If preoperative anesthetic was not used, a long-acting local anesthetic is infiltrated into the region of surgery for postoperative pain control. A cast is not used because it will restrict the nerve micro motion and may cause fibrosis.

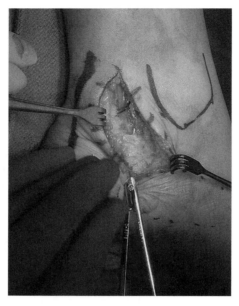

Fig. 4. Superficial retinaculum. Note the hemostat plantar to the sureficial retinaculum of the adductor muscle belly. This retinaculum is incised to allow the adductor muscle belly to be retracted to access the deep retinaculum, which makes up the medial plantar, lateral plantar, and calcaneal tunnels.

Instead, a bulky Sir Robert Jones-style dressing is placed with light compression. This needs to be bulky enough to restrict more than 5 degrees of motion in either dorsal or plantar motion. A temporary compression ace-wrap can be placed in the immediate post-operative period to limit the hyperemic reaction that follows the deflation of the tourniquet. This is typically removed in the recovery room about 30 minutes post surgery.

The patient is instructed to place no weight on the surgical foot and to use crutches. In case of poor balance, the heel may be placed on the ground and a walker may be used for stability as necessary. For the first 5 days following surgery, the posterior claf should be elevated and iced.

The patient is seen at 5–7 days for a wound check. The bulky dressing is removed and a small dressing is applied with a light compression wrap and an aircast ankle stabilizer. The patient is instructed to begin simple dorsiflexion and plantarflexion motion of the ankle for 10–20 minutes two times per day, with motion to the point of minimal pain. There should be no severe pain to motion noted by the patient. At 2–3 weeks, sutures are removed and ambulation in a tennis shoe with or without the use of the aircast is begun. A comprehensive physical therapy program is initiated; this is discussed in more detail in a subsequent article in this Clinics issue by Bond and colleagues. The patient may begin exercise and full activity as tolerated by 2–3 months post surgery. It is essential to explain to the patient that

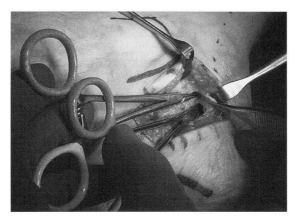

Fig. 5. Distinct medial and lateral plantar tunnels. Note the hemostats placed in the medial and lateral plantar nerve tunnels and the dividing retinacular branch. The retinaculum over each nerve is divided and the central dividing retinaculum is excised to make one large free tunnel. The index finger should easily fit into the arch of the foot after a full release.

tingling and pain may actually increase following surgery and that the numbness and pain may take up to 1 year to resolve while the nerve fibers begin to regenerate and the axonal flow returns to more normal levels.

Surgical results

Reported success rates after tarsal tunnel release with tibial nerve decompression have varied in the literature from 75%–91% [14]. The authors have achieved improved results after modifying their technique to include a more extensive and distal release of the posterior tibial nerve and its branches. A simple release of the flexor retinaculum is often not sufficient to achieve an adequate tarsal tunnel release, although this does depend on the specific etiology.

In 2003, Sammarco and Chang [14] reported on 75 surgical cases, with preoperative clinical findings and positive electrodiagnostic studies that confirmed the diagnosis of tarsal tunnel syndrome. After an average follow-up of 58 months, they reported that patients who had a pre-operative Maryland Foot Score of 61/00 that improved to 80/100 after surgery. They also found better results in patients who had symptoms for shorter than 1 year; these patients did better than patients who had tarsal tunnel syndrome for longer than 1 year.

Endoscopic tarsal tunnel release has been described in the literature, is designed to limit the trauma to the patient, and to produce a faster recovery time [20]. In their update paper in 1996, Day and Naples [20] related five cases, all with excellent results.

The authors believe the endoscopic approach relies upon a strong clinical suspicion that the only pathology is a tight flexor retinaculum. It is difficult to make this assumption, even with the use of imaging studies and electrodiagnostic exam. It is important to perform a release of the flexor retinaculum, also to explore the tarsal tunnel, and release the nerve more distally, through the abductor canal.

Cracchiolo and Pfeiffer [21] presented their surgical results after tarsal tunnel decompression which included long-term follow-up (average 31 months) on 30 patients. They reported only a 44% success rate defined as a good or excellent result. They noted 38% were clearly dissatisfied with the procedure. They suggested that the best indication to perform surgery for tarsal tunnel syndrome is the presence of a space-occupying lesion, and that this etiology produces the most predictable surgical outcome [21].

Nagaoka and Satou [22] confirmed this assertion. They presented the results of 30 feet that had tarsal tunnel secondary to the presence of a ganglion. They related that the mass was palpable in 28 of the 30 patients, and ultrasound was used to confirm or make the diagnosis in select patients. Surgical results were favorable for all 29 patients who underwent surgery [22].

Handrix and colleagues [17] discuss chronic intractable heel pain and present the surgical results of nerve decompression. Surgery included decompression of the posterior tibial, medial and lateral plantar nerve, and the first branch of the lateral plantar nerve. The surgery produced positive outcome in 96% of the patients [17].

Summary

Although tarsal tunnel remains a difficult diagnosis and problem to treat, advances in the procedure have improved surgical outcomes. The advent of neurosensory PSSD testing or adjunct EMG/NCV testing has resulted in a more complete understanding of the level of entrapment.

Futhermore, surgical outcomes have dramatically improved with a more comprehensive release of the foot nerves in addition to the tibial nerve. Internal neurolysis facilitates a second level of nerve decompression in needed cases. Early motion prevents nerve scarring and soft tissue scar formation, and physical therapy protocols have made it possible for patients to return to ambulation with limited long- term down time.

Tarsal tunnel syndrome still remains a complex and often under-diagnosed or misdiagnosed condition that affects the foot and ankle. It is essential to keep this problem in mind when treating heel pain, posterior tibial pain, and pain at the arch or ball of the foot. A proper work-up, thorough treatment, and supportive care in physical therapy, can make it possible for anyone who suffers from tarsal tunnel syndrome to return to full and unrestricted activity with minimal to no pain.

References

[1] Pollock L, Davis L. Peripheral nerve injuries. New York: Paul Hobner; 1933. p. 484–93.

[2] Kopell HP, Thompson WAL. Peripheral entrapment neuropathies of the lower extremity. N Engl J Med 1960;262:56–60.

[3] Keck C. The tarsal tunnel syndrome. J Bone Joint Surg 1962;44(A):180–2.

[4] Lam SJS. A tarsal-tunnel syndrome. Lancet 1962;2:1354–5.

[5] Mendicino SS, Mendicino RW. The tarsal tunnel syndrome and its surgical decompression. Clin Podiatr Med Surg 1991;8(3):501–12.

[6] Dellon AL. Computer-assisted sensibility evaluation and surgical treatment of the tarsal tunnel syndrome. Adv Podiatr Med Surg 1996;2:17–40.

[7] DiGiovanni BF, Gould JS. Tarsal tunnel syndrome and related entities. Foot Ankle Clin 1998;3(3):405–26.

[8] Persich G, Touliopoulos S. Tarsal tunnel syndrome. Available at: www.emedicine.com/orthoped/topic565.html.

[9] Lau JTC, Daniels TR. Tarsal tunnel syndrome: a review of the literature. Foot Ankle Int 1999;20(3):201–8.

[10] Dellon AL, Mackinnon SE. Tibial nerve branching of the tarsal tunnel. Arch Neurol 1984; 41:645.

[11] Havel PE, Ebraheim NA, Clark SE, et al. Tibial branching in the tarsal tunnel. Foot Ankle 1988;9:117–9.

[12] Reade BM, Longo DC, Keller MC. Tarsal tunnel syndrome. Clin Podiatr Med Surg 2001; 18(3):395–408.

[13] Belding RH. Neurilemoma of the lateral plantar nerve producing tarsal tunnel syndrome: a case report. Foot Ankle 1993;14:289–91.

[14] Sammarco GJ, Chang L. Outcome of surgical treatment of tarsal tunnel syndrome. Foot Ankle Int 2003;24(2):125–31.

[15] Mann RA. Letter to the editor. Foot Ankle Int 2000;21(7):616–7.

[16] Trepman E, Kadel NJ, Chisholm K, et al. Effect of foot and ankle position on tarsal tunnel compartment pressure. Foot Ankle Int 1999;20(11):721–6.

[17] Henrix C, Jolly GP, Garbalosa JC, et al. Entrapment neuropathy: the etiology of intractable chronic heel pain syndrome. J Foot Ankle Surg 1998;37(4):273–9.

[18] Pecina M. Letter to the editor. J Bone Joint Surg 2002;84A(9):1714–5.

[19] Kinoshita M, Okuda R, Morikawa J, et al. The dorsiflexion-eversion test for diagnosis of tarsal tunnel syndrome. J Bone Joint Surg 2001;83-A(12):1835–9.

[20] Day FN, Naples JJ. Endoscopic tarsal tunnel release: update 96. J Foot Ankle Surg 1996; 35(3):225–30.

[21] Pfeiffer W, Cracchiolo A. Clinical results after tarsal tunnel decompression. J Bone Joint Surg 1994;76-A(8):1222–30.

[22] Nagaoka M, Satou K. Tarsal tunnel syndrome caused by ganglia. J Bone Joint Surg 1999; 81B(4):607–10.

ELSEVIER
SAUNDERS

Clin Podiatr Med Surg
23 (2006) 611–620

CLINICS IN
PODIATRIC
MEDICINE AND
SURGERY

Anterior Tarsal Tunnel Syndrome

Lawrence A. DiDomenico, DPM[a],*,
Eric B. Masternick, DPM[b]

[a]Ohio College of Podiatric Medicine, Department of Surgery,
Northside Medical Center, 500 Gypsy Lane, Youngstown, OH 44505, USA
[b]Beeghly Medical Park, Suite 104, 6505 Market Street, Youngstown, OH 44512, USA

Several nerve compression syndromes have been described in the foot and ankle literature. The most frequently reported syndrome is the posterior tarsal tunnel syndrome, which is compression of the posterior tibial nerve.

Entrapment neuropathy of the deep peroneal nerve, also recognized as the anterior tibial nerve, typically occurs at the anterior ankle and dorsal foot. It provides sensory innervation of the skin between the first and second digit of the dorsal aspect of the foot [1]. Compression of the nerve, which anatomically is inferior to the extensor retinaculum, is commonly referred to as anterior tarsal tunnel syndrome. Although rare, this syndrome remains poorly diagnosed among clinical problems. Kopell and Thompson [2] first described deep peroneal nerve entrapment in 1963. In 1968, Marinacci [3,4] named the entity anterior tarsal tunnel syndrome and established the electrodiagnostic technique to assist in the diagnosis. The deep peroneal is the main branch of the common peroneal nerve. The common peroneal nerve passes the peroneal tunnel at the fibular neck, and then divides into the superficial, deep, and recurrent peroneal nerves. The deep peroneal nerve runs into the anterior compartment of the lower extremity between the anterior tibial, extensor hallucis longus muscles, and tendons. The deep peroneal nerve innervates the anterior tibial, extensor digitorum longus, extensor hallucis longus, and peroneus tertius muscles. At the ankle joint, it travels under the inferior extensor retinaculum and divides into two terminal branches: the lateral branch which innervates the extensor digitorum brevis muscle, and the medial cutaneous branch which is responsible for sensation between the first and second toes [5].

Anterior tarsal tunnel syndrome is frequently characterized by pain, weakness, and sensory changes of the foot and ankle. Chronic biomechanical mal-alignment, acute trauma, a direct blow, a soft tissue mass, bony

* Corresponding author.
  E-mail address: LD5353@AOL.com (L.A. DiDomenico).

exostosis, and tight shoe gear are common etiological factors that lead to anterior tarsal tunnel syndrome. Severe and chronic ankle sprains can cause unwarranted traction on the deep peroneal nerve which leads to symptoms consistent with anterior tarsal tunnel syndrome. Entrapment of the proximal portion of the deep peroneal nerve can lead to atrophy and weaken the anterior musculature. Entrapment of the distal portion of the deep peroneal nerve can produce first interspace sensory deficit and paresthesia. According to the literature, the most common cause of this compression is repetitive compressive trauma from tight shoe straps or high heel shoes (Figs. 1 and 2) [5]. Anterior tarsal tunnel syndrome has been reported with association of edematous lower extremities. Abdul-Latif and colleagues [6] reported a case of anterior tarsal tunnel syndrome secondary to edema in the post partum period. The diagnosis of anterior tarsal tunnel syndrome is made based on comprehensive knowledge of the anatomy linked with the appropriate history and physical examination findings. Treatment varies from non-operative care to surgical release of the nerve and decompression [7].

Anatomy

The deep peroneal nerve arises as a branch of the common peroneal nerve which courses around the neck of the fibula. The deep peroneal nerve enters the anterior compartment of the leg after it passes deep to the peroneus longus muscle and then flows obliquely forward beneath the extensor digitorum muscle. It then travels distally along the anterior surface of the interosseous membrane. In the upper one-third of the leg, the deep peroneal nerve is located between the extensor digitorum longus and the anterior tibialis muscles, and passes inferior to the extensor hallucis longus tendon in the lower one-third of the leg. The nerve is lateral to the anterior tibial artery and between the extensor hallucis longus and the extensor digitorum longus tendons, just proximal to the ankle joint. It then commonly divides into medial and lateral terminal branches about 1.3 cm above the ankle joint [8,9].

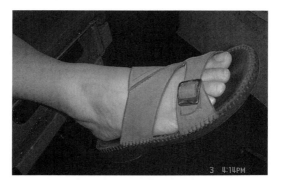

Fig. 1. A strap from a sandal can cause compression over the deep peroneal nerve.

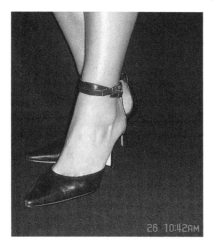

Fig. 2. A strap from a dress shoe can cause compression to the anterior ankle.

The medial branch travels to the first intermetatarsal space along the course of the dorsalis pedis artery which is located between the extensor hallucis longus tendon and the medial border of the extensor hallucis brevis muscle, where it pierces the deep fascia at the first webspace. At this point, it divides into two cutaneous nerves, which supply the medial aspect of the hallux and the lateral aspect of the second digit [8,9].

The lateral branch becomes enlarged just inferior to the extensor digitorum brevis muscle to supply a motor branch to the muscle and then gives off terminal branches to supply sensation to the second, third, and fourth metatarsophalangeal joints [8,9]. An accessory motor branch from the superficial peroneal nerve has been found to innervate the extensor digitorum brevis in 19% to 28% of subjects [10–13].

As the nerves and tendons pass along the ankle, they pass at almost a 90° angle; to prevent bowstringing they are held in place by retinacula. The superior extensor retinaculum is poorly definable and extends from the distal aspect of the fibula to the anterior tibial crest and medial malleolus. The inferior extensor retinaculum has a Y-shaped configuration, which originates from the sinus tarsi and tarsal canal laterally and then inserts into the medial malleolus proximally and the medial cuneiform and navicular distally [8,9].

Clinical findings

Anterior tarsal tunnel syndrome most commonly presents with altered sensations such as hyperesthesia, hypesthesia in the dorsal first web space, paresthesia which radiates to the first web space, pain upon palpation of the deep peroneal nerve in the entrapped area, pain in the dorsum of the foot, loss of ability to hyperextend the digits and hallux, and a vague burning sensation in the distribution of the deep peroneal nerve [9,14]. Wasting of the extensor hallucis brevis and extensor digitorum brevis muscles may be present. Two- point discrimination in the numb region may also be reduced with entrapment [1]. Tenderness to pressure along the deep peroneal nerve will be present either beneath the inferior extensor retinaculum, or distally at the apex of the first and second web spaces at the metatarso-cuneiform joints.

Pain associated with anterior tarsal tunnel syndrome usually worsens with activity and may reside with rest. Nighttime pain is also common because the foot is held in plantarflexion which causes the deep peroneal nerve to be at its stretched position [9,15]. Schon and coworkers [16] studied anterior tarsal tunnel syndrome in athletes and found that repetitive dorsal trauma, such as in soccer players, will cause similar symptoms. Repetitive trauma was also caused by bars used for sit-ups, and keys placed beneath the tongue of a running shoe (Fig. 3)[16].

As with any entrapment neuropathy, sensory abnormalities appear in the cutaneous distribution of the deep peroneal nerve. A Tinel's sign is elicited by percussion at the extensor hallucis brevis muscle. The patient's symptoms may be recreated by plantarflexion and inversion of the foot [9,14]. Confirmatory electrodiagnostic testing is recommended. In 28% of the patients there is the possibility of an accessory deep peroneal nerve which branches off of the superficial peroneal nerve [15].

Differential diagnosis

When a patient presents with anterior foot pain, along with anterior tarsal tunnel syndrome, the differential diagnosis may include lumbosacral nerve root impingement, peripheral neuropathy, medial tarsal tunnel syndrome, Morton's neuroma, superficial nerve entrapment, gout, peripheral vascular disease, bony ankle impingement, and ankle sprain or fracture [15].

It is very important to distinguish between an entrapment of the superficial peroneal nerve and the deep peroneal nerve. The superficial peroneal

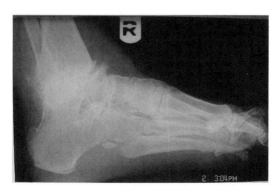

Fig. 3. Radiograph shows tibial talar exostosis, which causes compression and anterior tarsal tunnel syndrome.

nerve innervates the dorsum of the foot cutaneously, and percussion of the intermediate dorsal cutaneous branch will elicit paresthesia, pain, and a Tinel's sign. Compression of the superficial peroneal nerve will not result in muscle atrophy as would compression of the deep peroneal nerve [14].

Compression of the common peroneal nerve proximally at the level of the fibular neck must also be considered in the differential diagnosis of anterior tarsal tunnel syndrome. Compression of this nerve would result in weakness of the peroneals, anterior tibial, and extensor digitorum longus muscles. Even more proximal would be an L5 to S2 radiculopathy, which would produce more sensory impairment in a dermatomal pattern, and loss of Achilles tendon deep reflex [14,15,17].

Electromyographic and nerve conduction studies can determine if there is more proximal nerve involvement, such as lumbar radiculopathy, or if a polyneuropathy is present. The point of stimulation is proximal to where the entrapment is suspected and a delayed motor latency > 5 ms compared with the contralateral side, represents entrapment of the motor branch [18]. These results should be taken with caution and correlated with clinical findings because chronic or acute denervation of the extensor digitorum brevis is common in many other peripheral nerve diseases and also in some normal subjects.

Etiology

Anterior tarsal tunnel syndrome is caused by a compression of the deep peroneal nerve either by the extensor hallucis longus tendon or the inferior extensor retinaculum. The nerve lies in an unprotected area of the foot and ankle and could also be compressed by the talar head as the nerve passes over the talonavicular joint area (Fig. 4) [1].

Anything that can cause abnormal compression of the deep peroneal nerve can be a cause of the syndrome including fracture, subluxations, soft tissue masses, and wearing high-laced boots. The deep peroneal nerve is placed under maximal stretch while the foot is in plantarflexion and the digits are extended: the position of the foot in high-heeled shoes worn by women [18]. This maximal stretch would also support the clinical findings that anterior tarsal tunnel syndrome is worse at night in some patients because of the position of the foot during sleep.

A biomechanical etiology of anterior tarsal tunnel syndrome described in the literature is a result of a rigid forefoot valgus deformity associated with a plantarflexed first ray, which is compensated for by subtalar supination and midtarsal joint inversion [19].

Treatment

To treat anterior tarsal tunnel syndrome, conservative measures should be attempted first. Non-surgical treatment consists of removing external pressures that cause compression or traction on the deep peroneal nerve.

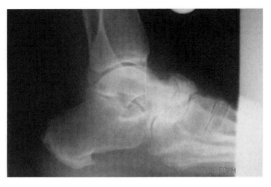

Fig. 4. Radiograph shows talar navicular exostosis, which causes compression to the deep peroneal nerve.

Initial non-operative treatment consists of patient education, pharmaceutical agents, local injections, physical therapy, and patient lifestyle modifications such as shoe wear and activity. Orthotics or accommodative shoes can help decrease the pressure over the nerve [20]. Different shoe gear, alternative lacing techniques, or appropriate padded areas may also accommodate the nerve. Patients who have recurrent ankle sprains and loss of proprioception might benefit from physical therapy to strengthen the peroneal muscles and improve ankle joint proprioception. Anticonvulsant or tricyclic antidepressant medications can diminish the neuritis and can be used in conjunction with pressure relieving treatment.

Conservative management of anterior tarsal tunnel syndrome has been successful. Abdul-Latiff and colleagues [6] reported a case in which post partum edematous lower extremities caused anterior tarsal tunnel syndrome and the patient responded well to leg elevation and diclofenac. Gessini and coworkers [21] reported on four cases of anterior tarsal tunnel syndrome: three patients responded to local steroid injection; the fourth patient responded to shoe gear modification. Non-steroidal anti-inflammatory medication and local infiltration of steroids at the site of entrapment are common traditional modalities used. When acute trauma is related to the deep peroneal nerve, immobilization is required. When neuropathy is associated with localized chronic edema, treatment of the primary condition may be effective.

If non-surgical efforts fail to relieve the symptoms, nerve decompression should be performed. The patient is placed in the supine position and receives either general or spinal anesthesia. The extremity is prepped in the usual sterile fashion and a mid-thigh tourniquet is used for hemostasis. A longitudinal or lazy S-shaped incision is made along the proximal ankle and extends to the base of the first and second tarsal-metatarsal joints. The incision is deepened between the extensor digitorum longus and extensor hallucis longus tendons. The nerve proximal to the cruciate crural

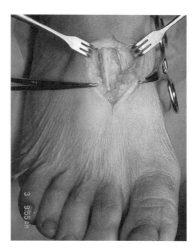

Fig. 5. An intra-operative view of the deep peroneal nerve after resection of the extensor hal-lucis brevis tendon.

ligament should be visible, and care should be taken to recognize the inter-mediate (Lemont's) and medial dorsal cutaneous nerves superficially [22]. The superiomedial and inferiomedial limbs of the inferior extensor retinac-ulum are divided. The deep peroneal nerve and the anterior tibial artery are identified. The deep peronel nerve along with the lateral and medial branches is neurolysed. An exploration for osteophytes, scar tissue, lesions and masses is performed and removed if located. The portion of the extensor hallucis brevis tendon that crosses the deep peroneal nerve is bovied and resected (Fig 5). Using microsurgical instruments and technique, the epi-neurium is opened. If there is intraneural fibrosis present, an internal

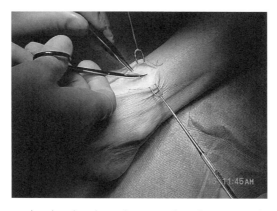

Fig. 6. An intra-operative view that shows decompression of a more proximal entrapment site.

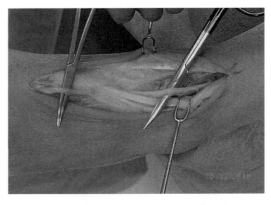

Fig. 7. An intra-operative view of the deep peroneal nerve after decompression proximal and distal. Note the extensor hallucis longus crossing over the nerve.

neurolysis is performed. The incision is closed with interrupted inradermal absorbable sutures and the skin is closed with staples.

For patients who have only a distal entrapment, an incision is made between the bases of the first and second metatarsals and extends proximal approximately 4 cm (Fig. 6). The incision is deepened into the subcutaneous tissues and the adjacent branches of the superficial peroneal nerve are acknowledged. The fascia is incised and the extensor hallucis brevis tendon is found crossing over the nerve. The tendon is bovied and a portion of the tendon is resected (over the nerve) and retracted. At this point the deep fascia is identified which causes pressure on the underlying nerve. The bony structures must be examined for osteophytes and, if any are present, resected. A release of the deep fascia proximally is performed and an internal neurolysis of the deep peroneal nerve is performed using microsurgical instruments and technique as indicated (Fig. 7). The incision is closed with interrupted inradermal absorbable sutures and the skin is closed with staples.

Postoperatively, the patient is injected with 10 mL of 0.5% marcaine along the incision. Adaptic, gauze, kerlex, and ace bandage are used from the metatarsal heads to the tibial tubercle for dressings. Early non-weight-bearing, range-of-motion exercises are encouraged. Patients should not bear weight for 2 weeks. The sutures are removed at 2 weeks and physical therapy is initiated.

Summary

Symptoms of anterior tarsal tunnel syndrome include a shock-like pain to the dorsal aspect of the foot, sensory loss, paresthesia in the first interspace, and possible atrophy of the extensor digitorum brevis muscle [23]. The cause of the syndrome is compression of the deep peroneal nerve in the anterior tarsal tunnel. There is very minimal soft tissue coverage at this anatomic site which leaves this area relatively unprotected. The site of entrapment can be at the superior edge of the inferior extensor retinaculum, over bony prominences of the dorsal medial tarsal bones, or under the extensor hallucis brevis tendon. Typical complaints heard from patients consist of vague neuritic aching pain of the foot and ankle. Numbness may or may not be present in the first web space. Atrophy of the extensor digitorum brevis muscle may be present if the nerve entrapment is proximal and involves the deep peroneal nerve motor branch. The nerve entrapment can be caused from external or internal compression. External compression is typically caused from contusion of the foot and ankle, tight boots, shoes, laces, or any pressure along the nerve. Bony lesions, soft tissue masses, scar tissue, or trauma that has initiated traction injuries to the local nerve can cause internal compression. The differential diagnosis of these indistinguishable symptoms is immense. The diagnosis is based on patient history and physical examination. Tinel's percussion sign is typically present at the site of the nerve entrapment. Injection therapy with a local anesthetic at the site of entrapment or proximal can help the physician make a diagnosis. Nuerosensory testing, nerve conduction studies, and electromyograms can be used to assess for nerve disorders or a more proximal nerve involvement. Nerve conduction studies in the lower extremity have a relatively high error rate; therefore, a negative study does not eliminate the diagnosis of nerve dysfunction.

There are non-surgical and surgical treatment options. Initially, non-operative measures should be attempted to reduce or remove the external compression along the anterior aspect of the foot and ankle. Other non-surgical options are shoe modifications, and cortisone injections with or without local anesthetics. Physical therapy can be provided to strengthen a weak ankle to prevent ankle instability.

If conservative management fails to relieve the patient's symptoms, surgical decompression of the entrapped nerve can be performed. The deep peroneal nerve is released from compressive forces in the entrapment site. This can be performed at the more proximal level at the extensor retinaculum or more distally at the level of the tarsal metatarsal site.

References

[1] Liu Z, Zou J, Zhao L. Anterior tarsal tunnel syndrome. J Bone Joint Surg Br 1991;73:470–3.
[2] Kopell HP, Thompson WAL. Peripheral entrapment neuropathies of the lower extremity. N Engl J Med 1960;262:56–60.
[3] Marinacci AA. Applied electromyography. Philadelphia: Lee & Febiger; 1968.
[4] Marinacci AA. Neurological syndromes of the tarsal tunnels. Bull LA Neurol Soc 1968;33: 90–100.
[5] Akyiiz G, Yilmar IT. Anterior tarsal tunnel syndrome. Electromyogr Clin Neurophysiol 2000;40:123–38.
[6] Abdul-Latif MS, Clarke S. Anterior tarsal tunnel syndrome in the post partum period. Int J Obstet Anesth 2001;10(1):75–6.

[7] Baumhauer JF. Entrapment of the deep peroneal nerve. Foot Ankle Clin N Am 1998;3(3): 427–37.

[8] Sarrafian S. The anatomy of the foot and ankle. Philadelphia: J.B. Lippincott; 1983.

[9] Adelman KA, Wilson G, Wolf JA. Anterior tarsal tunnel syndrome. J Foot Surg 1988;27(4): 299–302.

[10] Gutmann L. Atypical deep peroneal neuropathy in presence of accessory deep peroneal nerve. J Neurol Neurosurg Psychiatry 1970;33:453–6.

[11] Infante E, Kennedy WR. Anomalies branch of the peroneal nerve detected by electromyography. Arch Neurol 1970;22:162–5.

[12] Lambert EH. The accessory deep peroneal nerve: a common variation in innervation of extensor digitorum brevis. Neurology 1969;19:1169–76.

[13] Rubin M, Menche D, Pitman M. Entrapment of an accessory superficial peroneal sensory nerve. Can J Neurol Sci 1991;18:342–3.

[14] Kanbe K, Kubota H, Shirakura K. Entrapment neuropathy of the deep peroneal nerve associated with the extensor hallucis brevis. J Foot Ankle Surg 1995;34(6):560–2.

[15] Hirose CB, McGarvey WC. Anterior tarsal tunnel syndrome. Foot Ankle Clin N Am 2004;9: 255–69.

[16] Schon LC, Baxter DE. Neuropathies of the foot and ankle in athletes. Clin Sports Med 1990; 9:489–509.

[17] Kravette M. Peripheral nerve entrapment syndromes in the foot. JAPA 1971;61:457–72.

[18] Borges L, Hallett M, Selkoe B, et al. The anterior tarsal tunnel syndrome. J Neurosurg 1981; 54:89–92.

[19] Cangialosi CP, Schnall SJ. The biomechanical aspects of anterior tarsal tunnel syndrome. J Am Podiatry Assoc 1980;70:291–2.

[20] Hirose CB, McGarvey WC. Foot Ankle Clin N Am 2004;9:255–69.

[21] Gessini L, Jandolo B, Pietrangeli A. The anterior tarsal tunnel syndrome. J Bone Joint Surg 1984;66A:786–7.

[22] McGlamry ED. Acquired neuropathies of the lower extremities. Comprehensive textbook of foot surgery. 2nd edition. Baltimore (MD): Williams and Williams; 1992. p. 1106–10.

[23] Krause KH, Witt T, Ross A. The anterior tarsal tunnel syndrome. J Neurol 1977;217:67–74.

ELSEVIER
SAUNDERS

Clin Podiatr Med Surg
23 (2006) 621–635

CLINICS IN
PODIATRIC
MEDICINE AND
SURGERY

Surgical Decompression for Painful Diabetic Peripheral Nerve Compression and Neuropathy: A Comprehensive Approach to a Potential Surgical Problem

Babak Baravarian, DPM[a,b,c,*]

[a]UCLA School of Medicine, Los Angeles, CA, USA
[b]Foot and Ankle Surgery, Santa Monica/UCLA Medical Center, Santa Monica, CA, USA
[c]Foot and Ankle Institute Health Network, Los Angeles, CA, USA

The treatment of diabetic patients and the associated complications of diabetes have been extensively studied. Over the past several decades, the treatment of foot and ankle ailments in diabetic patients has dramatically shifted from conservative measures of "do not perform surgery" and "they will lose their limb anyway" to the present day thinking, which has taught us that diabetic feet are not very different from normal feet. The most common misconception with diabetic foot ailments has been that the loss of limbs is a result of severe vascular problems. However, with time, vascular issues in the diabetic foot have been found to be less problematic than previously suggested and less common than suspected. Often, the ulcer formation is the result of neuropathy and a lack of sensation. Following ulcer formation, the increase in blood supply necessary for healing may overwhelm the body and result in gangrene, infection, and potential limb loss.

What has been of interest is that the major cause of peripheral limb loss in the foot and leg of diabetic patients is a result of peripheral neuropathy and loss of protective sensation. The concept of protective sensation loss in the diabetic patient has always been noted to be irreversible, symmetrical, and progressive. However, a small number of interested researchers have

* Foot and Ankle Institute of Santa Monica, 2121 Wilshire Boulevard, Suite 101, Santa Monica, CA 90403.
E-mail address: bbaravarian@mednet.ucla.edu

0891-8422/06/$ - see front matter © 2006 Elsevier Inc. All rights reserved.
doi:10.1016/j.cpm.2006.05.003
podiatric.theclinics.com

been slowly and steadily attempting to show that there may be a compression syndrome associated with diabetic neuropathy that contributes to the pain and numbness of the foot, ankle, and lower leg. With time, there has been an increased interest in the surgical decompression of diabetic limbs to decrease pain and increase sensation. Although much controversy still exists, more and more doctors are beginning to understand the philosophy and potential for a chronic nerve compression of the diabetic limb.

Of interest to me was that during my residency, I spent a great deal of time with several hand surgeons. The surgeons performed a very large number of carpal tunnel releases in diabetic patients and never doubted that carpal tunnel may be possible in a diabetic patient. Now, when I think back to the nerves, they were often flattened and swollen beyond normal levels with internal scarring noted. The diabetic nerves often were far larger and more swollen than the nondiabetic cases. I met Dr Dellon discussing his peripheral nerve releases at a seminar while I was a resident and found the ideas interesting. He was definitely a very smart man, but I could not believe what he suggested could be true. I remember seeing many patients with diabetic foot pain who did not do well with conservative care or medication and I wondered what to do with them. After I spent some time in a fellowship program with Dr Dellon and the other 200 or so surgeons who perform the procedure for nerve decompression in diabetic patients and performing the procedure myself, I have come up with my own treatment protocols that I will share with you and also describe the surgery, the philosophy, and my beliefs. I truly feel that this is a revolutionary treatment with excellent potential, but I also think that it is essential to look at each case and weigh the benefits and risks of surgery versus conservative care. However, I truly feel that we have hit upon a potential treatment that may help millions of worldwide diabetic patients with relief of a chronic problem that has a very limited medical treatment at the present time. There have been many comments made that the majority of the studies performed have been from Dr Dellon and his faculty. This is not fully the case. As the initial and leading expert on the topic, Dr Dellon has dedicated his life to the topic and has done many basic research and clinical outcome studies on diabetic nerve release surgery. He has also instructed over 200 surgeons on the thinking, the testing, and the surgical outline for treatment of diabetic nerve pain and sensation loss. I know personally that he has dealt with a great deal of peer frustration as the leader in a new area, but with time, he has proven his ideas and has an international following at the present time. I also know that he has the cream of the crop of plastic surgeons working with him. His associates are all plastic surgeons with fellowship training in hand surgery or peripheral nerve surgery from the finest training programs. The question is why would a plastic surgeon with excellent training and a world of opportunity spend time on peripheral nerve surgery if the plastic surgeon thought it was not valid and revolutionary. What is most interesting is that the 200 or so surgeons performing diabetic nerve releases have formed a fellowship group and routinely add their surgical data to the fellowship patient outcome Web site.

With more than 2000 patient cases on the site from over 100 surgeons, the data are indisputable and difficult to miss. Overall, the results have been approximately 80% improvement in pain and 70% improvement in sensation among the study group patients with a positive Tinel over the involved nerve release sites. The results for pain relief and sensation restoration dip to 50% or 55% in the groups with no Tinel noted. This information is readily available for both surgeons and patients to review and is an attempt to take the fear and doubt out of this novel and exciting procedure. I hope that I will be able to help shed light on the ideas and basic research studies that have led to the thinking behind diabetic nerve decompression, the studies I perform to check the level of neuropathy, the conservative care that I try, and the surgical procedure. I urge those interested in performing such care to spend some time with a trained surgeon or with Dr Dellon to learn the subtle touches that make a world of difference to the surgical outcome.

Basic science research and one philosophy behind diabetic neuropathy

To take 40 years of research and sum it up in one or two sentences would not be very fair, but I feel it can be done. In 1973, Upton and McComas [1] initiated the theory of a double crush hypothesis suggesting that a nerve with serial limitations of axoplasmic flow may cause a more distal entrapment. In theory, diabetes is considered one cause of crush with a secondary local entrapment being the second cause. Although each of the crush factors may cause pain, the summation of multiple factors causes a far more symptomatic outcome than the parts. As a result, the local compression is a combination of a double crush existing due to a local entrapment in combination with a second crush factor, in this case being diabetes. However, the issue is far more involved when looked at in more detail.

Many studies have been performed on diabetic animal models. One of the first, in 1980, by Jakobsen and Sidenius [2] showed a decrease in axoplasmic flow with diabetes. Further studies by Tomlinson and Maher [3], Fink and colleagues [4], and Dahlin and colleagues [5] have confirmed the finding of decreased axoplasmic flow in diabetes. Many of the studies have involved use of rats and primates with streptozotocin-induced diabetes mellitus [6–8]. In such studies, the rat is made diabetic with the use of streptozotocin and following a period of time, a nerve biopsy and gait pattern changes are used to analyze the effect of diabetes on the peripheral nerves. Several rat studies have shown that the theory of a double crush phenomenon involving decreased axoplasmic flow as one crush and diabetes as a second crush [9] shows a chronic nerve compression of peripheral nerves as locations of possible impingement.

An additional finding suggested as a potential contribution to peripheral nerve compression in diabetic patients is the increased water content of the diabetic nerve as demonstrated by Jakobsen [10] in one study and Griffey and colleagues [11] in a second study. Several studies have shown that the increased size of the peripheral nerve as a result of increased water content may have caused chronic nerve compression at sites of anatomic narrowing in the upper and lower extremity [12–14]. The metabolic factors of diabetic neuropathy have been related to excess glucose conversion into intracellular sorbitol. The sorbitol is then thought to block the uptake of myoinositol leading to reduced sodium and potassium activity thought to be necessary for proper nerve conduction. A second point suggests that the increase of intracellular sodium results in paramodal demyelination [15]. With time, there is a decrease in axoplasmic flow eventually leading to axonal degeneration [16].

The vascular causes of diabetic neuropathy are still being extensively researched. It is clear to us that there is no small or large vessel disease associated with diabetic neuropathy [17–19]. However, there is a chance that axonal swelling may cause extraneural compression leading to axonal degeneration, demyelination, and nerve fiber loss [20–22].

The most common thought of a possible secondary cause of diabetic peripheral neuropathy is suggestive of possible biomechanical factors contributing to nerve entrapment at local compression regions. In the upper extremity, these sites would include the common peroneal nerve at the fibular head region; the tarsal tunnel and distal medial plantar, lateral plantar, and calcaneal tunnels at the medial ankle; and the deep peroneal nerve on the dorsum of the foot. Two causes have been associated with diabetic nerve compression syndrome. The first is compression at noted sites because of increased water content in the nerve resulting in axonal swelling, neural ischemia, and neuropathic symptoms [23]. Several studies have noted changes in the size and weight of the sciatic nerve in streptozotocin-induced rats. The second potential biomechanical cause of peripheral nerve pain is the loss of tissue elasticity and possible localized nerve impingement. Nonenzymatic binding of glucose to collagen in the epinuerium of the nerve may be a cause of decreased elasticity in the nerve [24]. With advanced glycosylation of the nerve, there is a loss of peripheral nerve gliding and increased tension about and along the nerve. This increase in tension may also cause a decrease in neural blood flow [25].

History and physical examination

The physical examination of peripheral nerve entrapment in the diabetic patient is quite straightforward. The standards that have been set by the many surgeons who perform the peripheral nerve releases in diabetic patients suggest that certain criteria must be met in the diabetic patient to increase the likelihood of positive results. The first and foremost point of importance is that the patient has pain or difficulty with ambulation and daily activity. In cases of numbness without pain, or in cases that respond well to oral neuropathy medications, surgery is not suggested as the risks may outweigh the potential positives.

In the history-taking process, the most common noted points are symmetrical numbness and pain that is debilitating. Often, the patient has tried several types of compounded foot creams and also been on multiple medications for neuropathy pain. Patients will often suggest that they have pain at night and have a difficult time with balance in the foot and ankle. They often have to take narcotic medication to calm the pain. Often they also feel that elevation and rest do not help the pain very much.

Physical examination should show good peripheral pulses including the femoral, popliteal, dorsalis pedis, and posterior tibial. If there is any question of peripheral circulation, transcutaneous oximetry or vascular Doppler testing with toe brachial index and segmental pressures may be used for additional information. Questionable cases of circulation should not have surgery until the circulation is completely checked and a clearance is obtained by a vascular surgeon. Foot musculature should be mature without severe weakness of all regions. Often, the common peroneal nerve entrapment results in weakness of the dorsiflexors of the foot including the anterior tibial and extensors. This may result in a shuffling gait pattern and weakness of the ankle and great toe to dorsiflexion strength. Hammering of the digits may also be noted owing to weakness of the intrinsics of the foot because of compression of the lateral plantar nerve branch at the ankle level. If surgery is being considered at the same time as ulcer closure, it is essential to make sure that the wound is clean with no gross signs of infection and no osteomyelitis as a cross contamination of the surgical sites is possible. In cases of gross infection, the wound or infection source should be treated before nerve release.

Nerve testing is quite simple to perform. In our hands, we avoid surgery on patients without a Tinel of the tibial and deep peroneal nerve and pain in the common peroneal nerve region. It is not to say that results cannot be positive in cases of negative Tinel, but the overall outcome is far better when signs of Tinel are noted. Nerve testing is performed with a tapping of the local nerve entrapment sites. The patient is asked if a tingling is noted with the tapping. A positive Tinel would suggest a proximal of distal tingling with tapping of the nerve. If a patient suggests that a different region is tingling than the site of sensory output for the local nerve, the test is not considered positive. If a negative Tinel is noted but a high index of suspicion is found and all other testing is positive, surgery is detailed to the patient with the level of positive outcome considered a 50% positive finding compared with 80% to 85% positive outcome with a positive Tinel finding.

Diabetic nerve testing

Although there has been a great deal of advancement in medicine for imaging of the musculoskeletal system, there has been little advancement in the diagnostic testing and potential imaging of the peripheral nerve system. Magnetic resonance imaging can be used to study potential space occupying lesions about the peripheral nerves and potential lumbar spine lesions. Computerized tomography also may be used to show potential boney impingement. Although both tests have a place in peripheral nerve studies, they are of little help in the diabetic patient. A recent study used ultrasonography of the peripheral nerves at sites of potential compression such as the tarsal tunnel to show reduction in the width of the nerve at the compression site and swelling of the nerve distal to the compression site [26]. This study provides hope for potential setup of ultrasound guidelines for assessment of peripheral nerve entrapment locations and the measurement of the nerve as a potential sign of entrapment syndrome.

Testing of the nerve for signs of peripheral neuropathy versus local compression have often relied on a nerve conduction velocity (NCV) and electromyelogram (EMG) testing. This sequence of testing potentially shows a decrease in the conduction velocity of the nerve along its course especially at locations of potential compression. Furthermore, supply of nerve impulse to local musculature may be potentiated with possible impingement resulting in slow to no muscle impulse. However, the testing has had severe limitations in its lower extremity uses. The rate of false negative data has been fairly inconsistent in the lower extremity and has shown problems with lower extremity testing. However, in a properly done test, the ideal test data will show distal axonopathy with decreased amplitude and decreased velocity and latency of the associated nerves with demyelination. The main use in our hands for EMG and NCV testing is to rule out potential lower back pain as a source of extremity pain. In cases of lower back pain with or without distal sciatic radiation, EMG and NCV testing can be used to evaluate radiculopathy.

A fairly new testing option that has been designed by Dr Dellon and his staff after years of trails is the pressure-specified sensory device (PSSD) (Sensory Management Services, LLC, Baltimore, MD). Studies comparing electrodiagnostic testing to PSSD testing have shown that the PSSD is at least as sensitive as electrodiagnostic testing studies [27]. The theory of the PSSD testing machine is quite simple. With increase in nerve compression, there is a loss of one- and two-point sensation threshold. This is similar to the Semmes Weinstein testing threshold (Dedham, MA) performed, however far more sensitive. Semmes Weinstein testing has shown that one point loss of protective threshold at 11.8 g would be similar to 90 g/mm^2 on the PSSD testing threshold [28,29]. Ulcer formation threshold is found to be at 30 g/mm^2 [30]. Therefore, by the time the Semmes Weinstein testing of protective threshold is positive, there is severe nerve damage and axonal loss. The essential improvement with the PSSD testing is that one- and two-point static and moving testing can be performed under controlled computer-driven settings. This allows better control of the amount of pressure and space between the two points needed to induce a sensation potential. With increase in one- and two-point static pressure findings, a deduction of possible nerve irritation versus mild entrapment is considered. If there is an increase in the width between the two points before sensation potential, axonal degeneration of the associated nerve is considered. The most common sites tested in the diabetic patient include the first web space representing the deep peroneal nerve region, the great toe pulp representing the tibial/medial plantar nerve region, the medial heel representing the tibial/calcaneal nerve region, and finally the lateral calf region representing the sciatic termination and common peroneal nerve region.

Our current diagnostic workup entails a neurosensory PSSD test in combination with local nerve ultrasound. Although we do not consider ourselves experts in ultrasound of peripheral nerves, we have gathered enough experience to begin routine ultrasounds of the peripheral nerves, especially the tibial nerve and its branches. The point of the ultrasound testing is to make sure there is no foreign mass in the region and check for the amount of compression on the nerve and the size of the nerve. Gliding of the nerve can also be checked but is far more difficult. Following ultrasound testing, peripheral PSSD testing is performed. Often, in diabetic patients, there are very poor results to preoperative testing but the level of neuropathy and nerve compression can be detailed.

Our current requirements for surgical consideration require a healthy patient who has no vascular issues, well-controlled diabetes levels, no gross infection, a positive Tinel, and positive PSSD testing. We may consider surgery on a patient with a negative Tinel test, but will explain that the results of surgery are not as successful compared with a patient with a positive Tinel.

Surgical procedure

The procedure may be done under local anesthesia with or without monitored anesthesia, or general anesthesia. As there is a need for thigh tourniquet use, general anesthesia is preferred for patient comfort. Following prepping of the limb, the thigh tourniquet is elevated and the procedure is begun. The first site for surgical decompression is the terminal sciatic nerve/common peroneal nerve. The leg is bent at the knee to a 90-degree angle and held by an assistant or a bolster. The nerve is easily palpated posterior and lateral to the fibular neck region. An incision is made along the lateral fibular neck extending from the posterior edge of the neck to the anterior peroneus longus region (Fig. 1). The incision is transverse in nature and measures 3 inches in length. Blunt dissection is carried through the soft tissue to the level of the covering fascia of the common peroneal nerve. Hemostasis is obtained with the use of bipolar cautery. The deep fascia is released over the common peroneal nerve with care being taken to avoid damage to the nerve. A good technique to use is to make a small incision into the fascia and then follow along the incision with a scissor releasing the fascia both posteriorly to the lateral edge of the knee and anteriorly to the level of the peroneus longus at which point the nerve passes deep to the fascia of the peroneus longus muscle. The lateral bands of the peroneus longus are divided along the course of the nerve and a small window is made at this region with dorsal and plantar release of the fascia fibers.

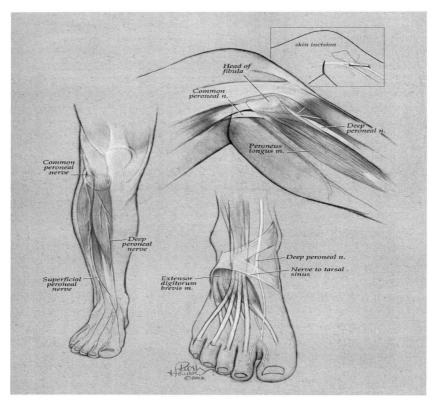

Fig. 1. Peroneal nerve release is performed with a transverse skin incision on the lateral fibular neck. The fascia over the common peroneal nerve and the lateral fascia of the peroneus longus muscle are released to decompress the common peroneal nerve. The deep peroneal nerve is released on the dorsum of the foot through a small linear incision. The key to the decompression is transection and removal of a small section of the extensor hallucis brevis tendon crossing the deep peroneal nerve on the dorsum of the foot. The retinaculum over the deep peroneal nerve is also freed. (Courtesy of A. Lee Dellon, MD, Baltimore, MD.)

Bipolar cautery of the fascia edges is performed to shrink the edge and prevent bleeding. If the nerve is found to be irritated by the lateral muscle branches of the peroneus longus muscle, these are also cauterized and released. The deep fascia of the peroneus longus is then released below the level of the common peroneal nerve. At this point, the index finger of the surgeon should easily glide along the released nerve and into the dorsum of the anterior shin. If there is an entrapment still noted, attention should be directed to the peroneus longus fascia and possibly the lateral aspect of the extensor digitorum longus muscle. Care should be taken when feeling the opening of the nerve and more distal release of the tunnel as the nerve will begin to give off muscular branches in this region, which must be protected. It is rare to require an epineural release of the common peroneal nerve, however a check of the nerve fibers should be performed. If extensive fibrosis is noted about the nerve, an epineural release is performed with micro dissection scissors. Copious lavage of the wound is performed and the incision is closed with the surgeon's choice of suture. We prefer to close the wound with an absorbable deep skin closure and skin staples. This allows for a more rapid allowance of movement of the region. Attention is then directed to the tarsal tunnel region.

The tarsal tunnel region surgery begins by marking common important landmarks. The medial malleolus, Achilles tendon, and navicular are all marked. The incision is linear to curvilinear incision centered between the medial malleolus and the Achilles tendon. The incision is also brought distally to the level of the medial abductor muscle belly at the point where the deep fascia covering the medial and lateral plantar nerve branches is thought to be present (Fig. 2). Careful dissection and cautery are performed to the level of the deep tarsal fascia. Often, the fascia over the tibial nerve is not found to be the site of greatest tightness. A small incision is made into the tibial retinacular fascia and careful scissor release of the tibial nerve is performed. The nerve is freed proximally to the point at which the index finger can easily glide along the nerve in a proximal fashion. Bipolar cautery of the edges of the fascia is performed. Care is then taken to identify the lateral cutaneous calcaneal nerve branch off the tibial nerve. This nerve is protected for lateral release. The superficial fascia of the abductor muscle belly is released and the muscle is distally and plantarly protected exposing the deep fascial tunnels of the medial, lateral, and calcaneal nerve branches. The tunnels are identified with a straight hemostat and the dividing fascial branch is also identified for release. The fascial tunnels are released along the line of each nerve branch. Care is taken to avoid damage to the venous plexus often found in the distal tunnel region along the medial arch region. Following release of the medial plantar and lateral plantar tunnels, the dividing fascial band between the two tunnels is released making one large tunnel that should allow the pinky or index finger to easily enter the arch and reach close to the the level of the navicular tuberosity. The calcaneal branch tunnel is then also released taking care to not injure the nerve as it traverses below the calcaneus. Bipolar cautery of the fascial tunnel edges is performed for as far along the tunnel as is visible and easily accessible. Any venous branches crossing and placing pressure on the tibial nerve or its distal branches are also released and cauterized. The tibial nerve is then checked for any endoneural thickening and, if found, microdissection release of the endoneurium of the nerve is performed. The region is lavaged and closed with the surgeon's choice of closure. Again, we prefer a nonabsorbable deep skin closure and staple skin closure. Attention is directed to the deep peroneal nerve region.

The deep peroneal nerve entrapment site is located on the dorsum of the foot in the region of the first and second metatarsal base/cuneiform region. The main culprit of entrapment in this region is the tendon of the extensor

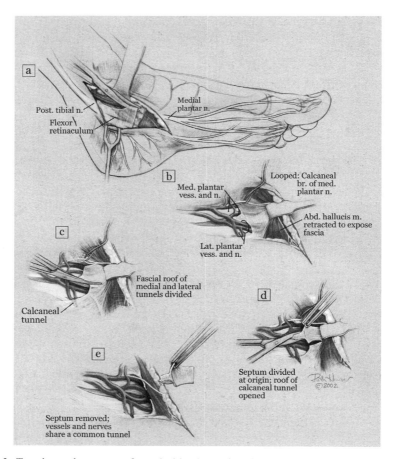

Fig. 2. Tarsal tunnel surgery performed with release of the flexor retinaculum (*A*), retraction of the abductor muscle belly and exploration of the deep retinaculum over the meidal and lateral plantar nerves and calcaneal branches of the tibial nerve (*B*). The three distinct tunnels of the medial plantar, lateral plantar, and calcaneal tunnels are freed (*C, D*) and the septum dividing the medial and lateral plantar tunnels are opened to make one large tunnel into the arch (*E*). (Courtesy of A. Lee Dellon, MD, Baltimore, MD.)

hallucis brevis, which has been shown to cross over the deep peroneal nerve and be a source of potential irritation [24] (Fig. 1). The deep peroneal nerve may also be pressured by the dorsal extensor retinaculum. A dorsal linear incision is placed over the region of the deep peroneal nerve centered about the first to second metatarso-cunieform joint. The incision is angled slightly lateral to medial from proximal to distal. The best way to find the exact location for the incision is to feel for the dorsalis pedis pulse before surgery, mark this region, and make an incision just medial to the dorsalis pedis. The incision is bluntly dissected through the deep tissues to the level of the extensor brevis tendon and retincular layer. Bipolar cautery is performed.

A section of the extensor tendon located over the nerve is removed. This section is commonly 2 cm in length. The retinaculum is then freed over the dorsal aspect of the nerve along its entire course. The retinaculum is usually 3 to 4 cm in length and easily freed with a scissor. Once the nerve is freed dorsally, the actual nerve is checked. Often there is a dell over the dorsum of the nerve at the region of the extensor tendon crossing with bulbous enlargement distal to this site. It is rare to require an endoneural dissection of the nerve and, in most cases, the nerve is found to not have severe internal scar formation. The region is lavaged and subcutaneous sutures are placed. Skin is closed with the surgeon's choice of material but again I prefer to use staples as they offer additional strength and allow for more rapid weight bearing.

The region is dressed with a bulky dressing that will allow slight movement but will not allow for extreme motion. Care is taken not to make the dressings very tight and to prevent severe compression across the nerve sites. A soft wrap cotton padding often used for Jones compression-style dressings is an excellent option. A mild compression ACE wrap is placed over the bulky soft padding for slight compression. No casting is performed.

The patient is allowed to touch his or her heel to the ground and is taught to use either crutches or a walker for balance and limited weight bearing. A wheel chair may also be used. The initial dressings are removed at 5 days and a wound check is performed. A light dressing is placed and the ankle is stabilized with an aircast-type brace. The patient is still to bear limited weight on the foot but is allowed to move the foot in a dorsal and plantar manner for 5 minutes per day with very slow motion. A subsequent visit is performed at the 3-week postsurgical period at which time staples or stitches are removed and physical therapy is started. Wound healing should be complete before removal of staples and initiation of therapy. The patient is allowed to return to normal shoes and walking without exercise walking for an additional month. The aircast brace may be worn for swelling control for an additional month at the desire of the patient.

The goal of therapy is multiple in nature. Initially, the goal is to calm swelling and prevent scar formation. Cross fiber and deep tissue massage, ultrasound, and laser therapy are initially used. Gentle and guarded motion is begun. Over time, physical therapy protocol begins for balance improvement and proper proprioception, balance, and comfortable ambulation. Overall, the period of therapy is often 1 to 2 months.

The patient is cleared for return to full activity at 2 to 3 months postsurgery. Often, the patient will feel less pain immediately after surgery and may or may not require pain medication or neuropathy medication for a period of 2 to 6 months postsurgery. Often, the neuropathy medication is tapered off in the initial 2 to 3 months postsurgery. It is not unusual to have patients feel complete relief of severe pain within days of surgery. However, in most cases, there is continued pain and tenderness for 2 to 6 months postsurgery at which point the nerve begins normal axonal transport and pain subsides.

Results of surgical decompression

Although the majority of surgical outcomes have been presented by A. Lee Dellon, MD, and his partners, this is somewhat to be expected as he is the innovator and developer of the procedure and has done the majority of physician training related to the surgery. Dellon initially presented his results in 1991 on 51 upper extremity and 31 lower extremity surgeries [31]. Electrodiagnostic testing was performed for the preoperative testing. Patients with positive local compression syndrome on testing showed 100% relief with surgery. Those with preoperative electrodiagnostic testing suggestive of neuropathy had 50% relief. When there was a finding of neuropathy and local compression, the results showed an improvement in 80% of patients.

Diabetic neuropathy cases have been less commonly reported than general nerve compression studies. Wieman and Patel [32] reported on 26 patients with diabetic neuropathy. An isolated tarsal tunnel release was performed on 33 legs. A significant improvement in pain was seen in 92% of patients while 72% showed an improvement in sensation. Two patients with a negative Tinel test preoperatively did not have any improvement after surgery leading the authors to conclude that a positive Tinel test is essential for good outcomes, while diagnostic testing did not seem to convey any form of optimal outcome potential.

Aszmann and colleagues [33] presented their results of nerve decompression on 31 nerves with 20 diabetic patients. Both upper and lower extremity decompression was performed and a therapist was blinded to the site of surgery and PSSD testing was performed for sensibility of the surgical versus the nonsurgical limb. Improvement in PSSD testing was noted on 69% of lower and 88% of upper extremities with worsening of neuropathy on the nonsurgical limb.

Dellon and colleagues [34] also presented results showing the importance of a Tinel sign in determining sensation restoration results in diabetic and nondiabetic neuropathy. In diabetic patients, the presence of a positive Tinel was noted to have a sensitivity of 88% and specificity of 50%. There was also a positive predictive value of 88% in showing good to excellent results in outcome prediction.

Caffee [35] also has reported on diabetic nerve release in the lower extremity involving diabetic patients. Thirty-six patients with 58 tibial nerve-release procedures were included in the study. Eighty-six percent of patients had significant pain relief after surgery. In patients with numbness as the main complaint, only 60% had improvement in initial complaint findings. Finally, none of the patients developed a foot ulcer postsurgery.

Biddinger and Amend [24] presented results of lower extremity triple site release of 18 patients involving 25 operative lower extremities. Fifteen of the patients had diabetic neuropathy while three had idiopathic neuropathy. Eighty percent of patients and 88% of legs with triple release were satisfied with the surgery. Pain was improved by an average of 4 points while numbness was improved by an average of 4.6 points. The study noted that when proper criteria including the presence of a Tinel's test over the entrapment sites is noted, pain can be relieved and sensation can be restored.

Rader [36] reported results of diabetic nerve release in 39 patients and 49 limbs in 2005. Preoperative and postoperative testing were performed by a technician who was blinded to the surgical site to prevent adjusted judgment. In all but six patients with bilateral nerve decompression, neuropathy medication was discontinued. A significant improvement of averaged one- and two-point sensation was noted postoperatively at 3 and 6 months with improvement of average levels noted at 6 months compared with 3 months. The visual analog scale (VAS) score was also noted to improve on average from a preoperative average of 8.72 to less than an average of 1 postoperatively. A very high level of patient satisfaction was also noted.

Valdevia and colleagues [37] also reported on 100 consecutive nerve decompression cares. Sixty of the patients were noted to have diabetes while 40 had noted idiopathic neuropathy. At 1 year of follow-up, 87% of patients with preoperative numbness reported improved sensation, 92% with preoperative balance problems reported improved balance, and 86% with a pain level of 5 or greater on the VAS scale before surgery reported improved pain level.

Summary

Diabetic nerve decompression is not for every patient. There is a definite learning curve to the surgery and recovery process and the surgeon must be available to the patient for concerns during the recovery period. The surgery itself is not very complex and can be mastered over time. Much like the idea that diabetic patients should not have surgery on their feet in the early seventies and the fact that diabetic charcot feet should not be reconstructed, especially in the early stages, the idea of nerve decompression in the diabetic patient is a foreign concept at the present time. The results, however, speak of a far different outcome. Pain relief and return to activity results have been excellent and, overall, the surgical decompression patients fair better in regard to ulcer formation and amputation risk than those without decompression. It is essential to select patients carefully and to make sure that the testing and examination findings discussed in this article are present before surgery.

With time, I believe that nerve decompression of the foot and leg in the diabetic patient will become as common as carpal tunnel release in the upper extremity is for the same group of patients. Education of the primary care physician and endocrinologist is essential to ensure proper and timely referral patterns before ulcer or foot infection. I truly believe that Dr Dellon and the rest of the world's peripheral nerve experts have dedicated their life to a worthy cause with the potential to help millions of suffering patients who have minimal to no answer for their symptoms from current medical care.

References

[1] Upton AR, McComas AJ. Hypothesis: the double crush in nerve entrapment syndromes. Lancet 1973;2:359–62.

[2] Jakobsen J, Sidenius P. Decreased axonal transport of structural proteins in streptozotocin diabetic rats. J Clin Invest 1980;66:292–7.

[3] Tomlinson DR, Maher JH. Defects of axonal transport in diabetes mellitus: a possible contribution to the etiology of diabetic neuropathy. J Auton Pharmacol 1984;4:59–72.

[4] Fink DJ, Purkiss D, Mata M. Alterations in retrograde axonal transport in streptozocin-induced diabetic rats. Diabetes 1987;36:996–1000.

[5] Dahlin LB, Meiri KF, Mclean WG, et al. Effects of nerve compression on fast axonal transport in streptozotocin-induced diabetes mellitus. Diabetologicia 1987;29:181–5.

[6] Mackinnon SE, Dellon AL, Hudson AR, et al. Chronic nerve compression: an experimental model in the rat. Ann Plast Surg 1984;13:112–20.

[7] Mackinnon SE, Dellon AL, Hudson AR, et al. A primate model for nerve compression. J Reconstr Microsurg 1985;1:185–95.

[8] O'Brien JP, Mackinnon SE, MacLean AR, et al. A model of chronic nerve compression in the rat. Ann Plast Surg 1991;26:430–5.

[9] Dellon AL, Mackinnon SE, Seiler WA. Susceptibility of the diabetic nerve to chronic compression. Ann Plast Surg 1988;20:117–9.

[10] Jakobsen J. Peripheral nerves in early experimental diabetes: expansion of the endoneurial space as a cause of increased water content. Diabetologia 1978;14:113–9.

[11] Griffey RH, Eaton RP, Sibbitt RR, et al. Diabetic neuropathy: structural analysis of nerve hydration by magnetic resonace spectroscopy. JAMA 1988;260:2872–8.

[12] Dellon AL. Operative technique for submuscular transposition of the ulnar nerve. Contemp Orthop 1988;16:17–28.

[13] Mackinnon SE, Dellon AL. Homologies between the tarsal and carpal tunnels: implications for surgical treatment in the tarsal tunnel syndrome. Contemp Orthop 1987;14:75–84.

[14] Dellon AL, Mackinnon SE. Radial sensory nerve entrapment in the forearm. J Hand Surg 1986;11A:199–205.

[15] Greene DA, Lattimer SA, Sima AF. Sorbitol phosphoinositides, and sodium-potassium-ATPase in the pathogenesis of diabetic complications. Semin Med Beth Israel Hosp Boston 1987;316(10):599–606.

[16] Fink DJ, Purkiss D, Mata M. Alterations in retrograde axonal transport in streptozotocin-induced diabetic rats. Diabetes 1987;36(9):996–1000.

[17] Strandness DE Jr, Preist RE, Gibbons GE. Combined clinical and pathologic study of diabetic and non diabetic peripheral arterial disease. Diabetes 1964;13:366–72.

[18] Barner HB, Kaiser GC, Willain VL. Blood flow in the diabetic leg. Circulation 1971;43:391–4.

[19] Conrad MC. Large and small artery occlusion in diabetics and nondiabetics with severe vascular disease. Circulation 1967;36:83–91.

[20] Dellon AL. Preventing foot ulceration and amputation by decompressing peripheral nerves in patients with diabetic neuropathy. Ostomy Wound Manage 2002;48(9):36–45.

[21] Gabbay KH. The Sorbitol pathyway and the complication of diabetes. N Engl J Med 1973; 288:831–6.

[22] Lundborg G, Rydevik B. Effects of stretching the tibial nerve of the rabbit: a preliminary study of the intraneural circulation and the barrie function of the perineurium. J Bone Joint Surg 1973;55B:390–401.

[23] Jakobsen J. Peripheral nerves in early experimental diabetes. Expansion of the endoneurial space as a cause of increased water content. Diabetologia 1978;14:113–9.

[24] Biddinger KR, Amend KJ. The role of surgical decompression for diabetic neuropathy. Foot Ankle Clin N Am 2004;9:239–54.

[25] Rydevik B, Lundborg G. Effects of graded compression on intraneural blood flow. J Hand Surg 1981;6A:3–12.

[26] Lee D, Dauphinee D. Morphological and functional changes in the diabetic peripheral nerve using diagnostic ultrasound and neurosensory testing to select candidates for nerve decompression. J Am Podiatr Med Assoc 2005;5:433–7.

[27] Tassler PL, Dellon AL. Correlation of measurements of pressure perception using the pressure specified sensory device with electrodiagnostic testing. J Occup Environ Med 1995;37:862–6.

[28] Dellon ES, Crone S, Mouery R, et al. Comparison of the Semmes-Weinstein monofilaments with the pressure-specifying sensory device. Restor Neurol Neurosci 1993;5:323–6.

[29] Dellon AL. Decompression of peripheral nerves for symptoms of diabetic neuropathy: pain management considerations. Pain Clin 2001;13:11–6.

[30] Tassler PL, Dellon AL. Pressure perception in the normal lower extremity and in the tarsal tunnel syndrome. Muscle Nerve 1996;19:285–9.

[31] Dellon AL. Treatment of symptomatic diabetic neuropathy by surgical decompression of multiple peripheral nerves. Plast Reconstr Surg 1991;99:679–87.

[32] Weiman TJ, Patel VG. Treatment of hyperesthetic neuropathic pain in diabetics: decompression of the tarsal tunnel. Ann Surg 1995;221(6):660–5.

[33] Aszmann OC, Kress KM, Dellon AL. Results of decompression of peripheral nerves in diabetics: a prospective, blinded study. Plast Reconstr Surg 2000;106:816–22.

[34] Dellon AL, Aszmann O, Tassler P. Outcome of surgical decompression of nerves in diabetics on incidence of ulceration and amputation. J Reconstr Micro 2003;19(5):350–5.

[35] Caffee HH. Treatment of diabetic neuropathy by decompression of the posterior tibial nerve. Plast Reconstr Surg 2000;106:813–5.

[36] Rader AJ. Surgical decompression in lower-extremity diabetic peripheral neuropathy. JAPMA 2005;5:446–50.

[37] Valdivia JM, Dellon AL, Weinand ME, et al. Surgical treatment of peripheral neuropathy: outcomes from 100 consecutive decompressions. JAPMA 2005;5:451–4.

ELSEVIER
SAUNDERS

Clin Podiatr Med Surg
23 (2006) 637–649

CLINICS IN
PODIATRIC
MEDICINE AND
SURGERY

Chemotherapy-Induced Neuropathy

Gedge D. Rosson, MD

Division of Plastic Surgery, JHOC 8th Floor, McElderry 8152-A,
601 North Caroline Street, Baltimore, MD 21287, USA

Medical oncologists have become more aggressive in their management of tumors by using protocols that call for higher or more frequent dosing of chemotherapy agents. As a result, podiatric and peripheral nerve surgeons will become increasingly involved in the care of patients who experience debilitating, painful neuropathy induced by chemotherapy [1]. Recent advances in cancer treatment have led to longer disease-free intervals for many tumors, and improving the quality of life of these patients will become progressively more imperative [2].

One of the most limiting factors of chemotherapy is frequently noted to be chemotherapy-induced peripheral neuropathy. The degree of the neuropathy and the amount of pain generated depends on the chemotherapy agent, the dose given at each dosing interval, and the cumulative dose [3]. Occasionally, peripheral neuropathy effects can become evident after a long delay following the cessation of the drug, referred to as "coasting" [4]. It is also well noted that the degree of peripheral neuropathy can be attributed to confounding factors such as pre-existing diabetes, alcohol neuropathy, hypothyroid neuropathy, or inherited neuropathies [4]. Additionally, the complications of chemotherapy are more common in elderly patients who have cancer [5].

Although peripheral neuropathy is one of the critical complications that affects quality of life, other common complications include myelosuppression, mucositis, cardio depression, and central neurotoxicity. Most often the underlying mechanisms are not completely understood; however, many use a final common pathway, including binding of the chemotherapeutic agent, like cisplatin or paclitaxel to tubulins in the axoplasm, or causing apoptosis of the dorsal root ganglion cells [6]. Although, there are many chemotherapeutic agents that do not cause peripheral neuropathy, some of the more well-known chemotherapy agents that frequently cause peripheral

E-mail address: gedge@jhmi.edu

0891-8422/06/$ - see front matter © 2006 Elsevier Inc. All rights reserved.
doi:10.1016/j.cpm.2006.04.009

neuropathy are widely used and include the vinca-alkaloids (vincristine), platinum compounds (cisplatin and oxaliplatin), and taxol compounds (paclitaxel).

There are also some older drugs that have gained new applications as chemotherapy agents, including suramin and thalidomide. Some new classes of chemotherapeutic agents are showing great promise for the treatment of malignancies; these include epithilones and proteasome inhibitors (Table 1).

In addition to drugs used to treat cancer, there are many other commonly used drugs that are now being reported to cause peripheral neuropathy, including statins, such as simvastatin (Zocor), and antibiotics, such as linezolid. It is also essential to consider that some cancers themselves can have paraneoplastic syndromes that mimic several forms of peripheral neuropathy. It has been shown that HIV can also have complications of peripheral neuropathy.

It is well reported in the literature that it is very difficult to assess patients for chemotherapy-induced neuropathy, especially because electromyogram (EMG) and nerve conduction studies do not detect early neuropathy [4]. Prominent investigators noted that in patients who have diabetic neuropathy, "nerve conduction studies do not reliably distinguish the presence or the absence of carpal tunnel syndrome in subjects with diabetes" [7]. They concluded that the diagnosis of carpal tunnel syndrome should be made independently from nerve conduction studies and based on clinical exam. Dellon provides an excellent review of electrodiagnostic testing versus neurosensory testing and describes how non-invasive neurosensory testing can be used to follow patients with nerve injuries over time [8]. I believe that chemotherapy-induced neuropathy can be followed with serial non-invasive neurosensory testing, such as two-point discrimination and static and moving pressure thresholds, in a similar fashion as diabetic neuropathy.

Vincristine

Vincristine is a vinca-alkaloid which binds to intracellular tubulins and causes dissociation of the microtubuli. This leads to edema of the fast- and slow-conducting axons [4]. Microtubular disorientation and axonal edema

Table 1
Examples of chemotherapy agents that commonly cause neuropathy

Drug type	Class	Agent	Trade name
Widely used	Vinca alkaloids	Vincristine	Oncovin
	Platinum compounds	Cisplatin	Platinol
	Taxanes	Paclitaxel	Taxol
Old drugs with new applications	Anti-protozoal	Suramin	
	Sedative hypnotic	Thalidomide	Thalomid
New classes	Epothilones	Ixabepilone	
	Proteasome inhibitors	Bortezomib	Velcade

have been shown in a rat model of vincristine [9]. This mechanism causes a dose-dependent, primarily sensory neuropathy [10]. The neuropathy of vincristine begins with paresthesias and pain of the hands and feet, and most often is accompanied with hyperesthesia. It can act like Guillain-Barré syndrome when given to children and to people who have hereditary neuropathies. Many symptoms are reversible after months or years but can be permanent, and "coasting" has been shown to occur with vincristine. Underlying subclinical neuropathies such as Charcot-Marie-Tooth disease can be made worse by the administration of vincristine. It is critical to rule out possible underlying neuropathies which could be exacerbated [11].

Cisplatin

Since 1978, peripheral neuropathy has been known to be a complication of cisplatin, a platinum-based compound that goes by the trade name of Platinol [12]. It is particularly effective against ovarian, testicular, and bladder cancers. This drug has other side effects, that include nephrotoxicity, otic toxicity, nausea, vomiting, and myelosuppression. The neuropathy is primary sensory, although can include mild motor involvement [13]. Most patients will improve with cessation of treatment, but some are permanently severely disabled [14]. A post-mortem study of nerves in patients who have cisplatin-induced neuropathy found that the platinum concentrations were significantly higher in the tumor, in the sural nerves, and the spinal ganglia compared with the brain, which suggests that cisplatin does not cross the blood-brain barrier [14]. The exact mechanism of cisplatin toxicity is not known, but it appears that cisplatin somehow disturbs the axoplasmic transport. Coasting occurs with cisplatin and cisplatin neurotoxicity progresses for weeks or months after cessation of dosing, which indicates the involvement of axoplasmic transport [15]. In an attempt to predict the peripheral neurotoxicity of cisplatin and paclitaxel, Cavaletti and colleagues [16] found that serial nerve growth factor samples did not help predict chemotherapy-induced peripheral neurotoxicity, but rather, they had to rely on clinical examination.

Oxaliplatin

Oxaliplatin is an alkylating agent that is also platinum-based. It goes by the trade name of Eloxatin. It inhibits DNA by forming interstrand and intrastrand cross-linking of the DNA. The exact mechanism of oxaliplatin-induced neuropathy is not known, but it may be related to oxaliplatin's affects on sodium channels by chelation of free calcium by the oxalate. Acute and chronic neuropathies are associated with oxaliplatin. The acute neuropathy is very common, occurs in 85% to 95% of all patients, and is usually self-limited [17]. The more problematic form is the chronic neuropathy that is caused by cumulative doses and is seen in patients who receive total doses > 540 mg/m^2 [18]. Fifty percent of patients show this chronic cumulative neuropathy when they have a cumulative dose of 1170 mg/m^2 [17]. The symptoms, fortunately, are mostly reversible, and after 12 months all patients have partially recovered; 40% of the patients have minimal residual neurologic symptoms [17].

Paclitaxel and docetaxel

Paclitaxel and docetaxel are taxol compounds. Paclitaxel and docetaxel go by the trade names of Taxol and Taxotere, respectively. The taxol compounds have been found to have excellent activity in ovarian, breast, lung, and head and neck cancers. The major toxicities include myelosuppression, hypersensitivity reactions, cardio-toxicity and neurotoxicity. Paclitaxel affects the aggregation of intracellular microtubules. The exact mechanism of neurotoxicity is not known, but studies have shown that there is a direct effect on Schwann cells, axonal loss, and disturbed cytoplasmic flow [19,20]. Sensory neuropathy is the most common neurotoxicity, although there have been some reports of motor neuropathies, autonomic neuropathies, central nervous system toxicities, and myopathic effects. It is suggested that there are both an axonopathy and a neuronopathy that result from the paclitaxel [21]. Docetaxel has been found to be beneficial in breast cancer, ovarian cancer, non-small-cell lung cancer, and head and neck cancer [22]. Docetaxel is also reported to cause a neuropathy, and cumulative dose levels > 600 mg/m^2 can cause a severe and disabling neuropathy [22,23]. Paclitaxel and docetaxel are quite similar in their structures and mechanisms of action, but clinical studies have shown differences in the toxicity profiles of the two drugs [24]. The general view of the medical community is reflected in a review article about the side effects of the treatment of breast cancer, which, when referring to the taxanes, stated "there are currently no effective means to prevent or treat taxane-induced neuropathy" [25].

Suramin

Suramin is an anti-protozoal used for African sleeping sickness (trypanosomiasis) and river blindness (onchocerciasis). It was developed originally in 1916, but it is now being studied for treatment of prostate cancer. It was found to be a potent reverse transcriptase inhibitor, although unfortunately it had limited benefits for HIV treatment. Currently, suramin has been found efficacious in the treatment of hormone-refractory or metastatic prostate cancer. Unfortunately, it has also been found to be neurotoxic. It does not cross the blood-brain barrier; therefore, the neurotoxicity has been limited to peripheral neuropathy. It is found to have a length-dependent axonal degeneration and also a demyelinating polyradiculoneuropathy. Clinically, it can have a Guillain-Barré syndrome type effect. Sural nerve biopsy has shown axonal degeneration and lymphocytic infiltration [26]. A rat model suramin neuropathy study showed that neuropathy developed within 2 weeks when rats were given high doses of suramin, and histology revealed evidence of axonal degeneration and axon atrophy. In patients who received low doses, the most severe effects were noted at 2 months. Lysosomal inclusion bodies in dorsal root ganglion Schwann cells were noted in electron microscopy. The conclusions in the rat model were that "suramin induced a length, dose, and time-dependent axonal sensory motor polyneuropathy associated with axonal degeneration, atrophy, and accumulation of glycol lipid lysosomal inclusions" [27].

Thalidomide

Thalidomide is approved by the Food and Drug Administration for treatment of erythema nodosum leprosum in Hansen's disease. It is now also being used for multiple myeloma and treatment of Waldenstrom's macroglobulinemia, myelodysplastic syndrome, renal cell carcinoma, and prostate cancer [28]. Thalidomide's main action is inhibition of angiogenesis [29]. In addition, it has been indicated in the inhibition of tumor cells by altering adhesion molecules, modulating cytokines, and increasing the number of $CD8^+$ T cells by immunomodulatory effects [30]. According to a discussion on treating Waldenstrom's macroglobulinemia, the primary reason to remove patients from therapy is neurotoxicity [31]. A recent review of thalidomide-induced neuropathy states that the mechanism is not entirely clear, but there is evidence of both a neuronopathy and an axonopathy [32]. There is some debate about whether the neurotoxicity is cumulative dose dependent. A prospective study in patients who have lupus erythematosus found no correlation between thalidomide cumulative dose and the appearance of peripheral neuropathy [33]. A clinical and neurophysiologic study of patients being treated with thalidomide for multiple myeloma, systemic lupus erythematosus, and monoclonal gammopathy of unknown significance found that there was a cumulative dose dependence, but only when the total dose was relatively high [34]. In a discussion of those two papers, Apfel [35] suggested that regardless of the dose, it is very important to review the patient's symptoms, perform regular neurologic examinations, and perform periodic screening of sensory nerve electrophysiology. Even though the phocomelia is the most serious and the most infamous toxicity of thalidomide, the most common complication in cancer patients today is actually the peripheral neuropathy, which can occur in more than 50% of patients [36].

Proteasome inhibitors

Bortezomib is the first member of a new class of chemotherapy agents. It goes by the trade name Velcade. Bortezomib is a potent, selective and reversible inhibitor of the proteasome, which ultimately leads to apoptosis of the cell. A phase I trial of bortezomib showed efficacy versus advanced tumor malignancies of many types [37]. Since then, there have been phase II studies which have shown efficacy of bortezomib against recurrent or metastatic sarcomas [38], relapsed and refractory myeloma [39,40], and relapsed or refractory B-cell non-Hodgkin's lymphoma [41]. The most common adverse effects of bortezomib therapy were thrombocytopenia, fatigue, peripheral neuropathy, and neutropenia [39,40]. Gastrointestinal side effects and fatigue were also noted [38,41]. Although it is very exciting that there is a new class of chemotherapeutic agents, in all of the studies to date, bortezomib has been found to be a significant cause of peripheral neuropathy in some patients. It is not known which mechanism causes the neuropathy, but in one study, at least one patient developed significant, grade 4 neuropathy while on a low dose of bortezomib [40].

Epithilones

The first member of this new class of chemotherapeutic agents is called ixabepilone. It is a microtubule-stabilizing agent which disrupts the microtubule function and leads to apoptosis. Ixabepilone is an epithilone B analog and has been shown to be effective in patients who were previously treated for advanced colorectal cancer [42], in metastatic and locally advanced breast cancer [43], and in patients who have progressive castrate metastatic prostate cancer [44]. The most common grade 3 and 4 toxicities noted were neutropenia, fatigue, neuropathy, hypersensitivity reaction, and gastrointestinal disturbances. The rates of the sensory peripheral neuropathy ranged from 3% [43] to 20% [42]. Much like the excitement over the proteasome inhibitors, we will probably see increased use of epithilones, which would result in more patients who have some form of peripheral neuropathy.

Other drugs

In a large review of the literature on statin-associated peripheral neuropathy, it is suggested that "statins should be considered the cause of peripheral neuropathy when other etiologies have been excluded" [45]. Although the incidence of statin-associated peripheral neuropathy is low, the very fact that statins are being increasingly used to treat hypercholesterolemia, and the target goals for total cholesterol level are constantly being lowered, it seems that this will become a more important cause of neuropathy. Statin-associated neuropathy should always be considered and discussed with the patient's primary care physician whenever a patient has neuropathy of unknown origin.

Linezolid is an antibiotic in the oxazolidinones class. Linezolid is known by the trade name Zyvox. It binds to the 70S ribosomal initiation complex and is used in the treatment of vancomycin-resistant enterococcus and also staphylococcus aureus, including methicillin-resistant staphylococcus aureus. Bressler and colleagues [46] found that linezolid was the cause of peripheral neuropathy in one of their patients and a review of the literature showed that other antibacterials, such as the quinolones, nitrofurantoin, and polymyxin B, may cause peripheral neuropathy [47].

HIV neuropathy

The human immunodeficiency virus has many effects, and besides causing an immune deficiency, it is well known to cause various neuropathies. Early on in the infection, there can be a seroconversion-related neuropathy that can manifest as facial nerve palsy or as Guillain-Barré syndrome [48]. As the disease progresses to its advanced stages, patients have been found to have evidence of chronic inflammatory demyelinating polyneuropathy and also diffuse infiltrative lymphocytosis syndrome. These patients are also at increased risk for co-infection with syphilis and hepatitis C, which can lead to their own neuropathies. In addition to neuropathies caused by HIV infection, the anti-HIV medications, such as stavudine, lamivudine, zalcitabine, and didanosine, can themselves cause a neuropathy [47].

Paraneoplastic syndromes

Not all neuropathies are caused by the chemotherapy agent itself. Actually, it has been shown that paraneoplastic syndromes that involve neuropathies can occur with several tumors, especially small-cell lung cancer and breast cancer [49–51]. Interestingly, the appearance of the paraneoplastic neurologic syndrome can often antedate the discovery of the malignancy. The most well-known paraneoplastic syndrome, Lambert-Eaton syndrome, involves the neuromuscular junction rather than the peripheral nerve. The most common peripheral nerve paraneoplastic syndromes are categorized into subacute sensory neuronopathy, acute demyelinating neuritis, chronic inflammatory demyelinating polyneuropathy (CIDP), neuropathy with paraproteinemia, and sensorimotor neuropathy. A comprehensive review of CIDP and its responsiveness to immunotherapy was published recently in the *New England Journal of Medicine* [52].

Medical management

Patients who require medical management of peripheral neuropathy from chemotherapy include those who have neuropathic pain. One of the mainstays of treatment today is gabapentin (Neurontin), which originally was shown to be extremely useful in the symptomatic treatment of painful neuropathy in patients with diabetes [53]. An excellent review of antineuralgic agents discusses the nociceptive pathways and etiology of neuropathic pain and then categorizes medications into modulators of peripheral sensitization, modulators of descending inhibitory pathways, modulators of central sensitization, and drugs with other mechanisms [54]. The modulators of peripheral sensitization include sodium-channel modulators, carbamazepine, phenytoin, topiramate, lamotrigine, topical lidocaine, mexiletine, and tricyclic antidepressants. The modulators of the descending inhibitory pathways include antidepressants such as the selective serotonin reuptake inhibitors, tramadol, and opioids. The modulators of central sensitization include gabapentin, levetiracetam, lamotrigine, ketamine, and dextromethorpham. Modulators with other mechanisms were capsaicin, levodopa/carbidopa, and non-steroidal anti-inflammatory drugs [54]. Another excellent review mentions these similar drugs and stresses the importance of initiating polypharmacy or multi-dimensional therapy [55]. When one drug gives partial relief, but an increasing or an escalating dose produces limiting side effects, then the dose should be decreased and other drugs added. A randomized, double-blind, placebo-controlled cross-over trial showed the combination of sustained-release morphine plus gabapentin "achieved better analgesia at lower doses of each drug than either as a single agent" [56]. A new drug called duloxetine (Cymbalta) has shown promise for neuropathic pain treatment, but there are no long-term studies.

Surgical management

Treating patients who have chemotherapy-induced neuropathy by using nerve decompression surgery in the upper and lower extremities is based on extrapolation from both published findings on decompression in patients with diabetic peripheral neuropathy, and on peripheral nerve decompression of chemotherapy-induced neuropathy in rats [57]. To date there have been anecdotal reports and one published study [58] that describes patients who improve from chemotherapy-induced neuropathy following decompression. It is believed that some of the putative causes of the peripheral neuropathies caused by chemotherapy may have similar mechanisms as diabetes-induced peripheral neuropathy and its increased susceptibility to chronic nerve compression [59,60].

Two studies have shown that decompression of the various nerves in the distal limbs of diabetic rats can reverse the functional effects of the diabetic neuropathy in those rats [61,62]. The rat model that shows diabetic nerves are susceptible to chronic compression gives us an early clue [59]. This concept is discussed in papers on diabetic neuropathy, which stress that overlying compressions should be diagnosed and that recommend decompressive surgery [63,64]. Several studies have been published that document the results of decompressing peripheral nerves for treatment of symptomatic diabetic neuropathy, in both the upper and lower extremities [65–71]. One of the main positive prognostic signs to look for in both diabetic and non-diabetic neuropathy is the presence of a positive Tinel-Hoffman sign [72]. In fact, in a retrospective analysis of 50 patients with diabetes who had surgery on only one limb, there were 12 ulcers and 3 amputations in the contralateral limbs at an average of 4.5 years from the date of surgery. This implies that the decompression of the nerves in patients who have diabetic neuropathy and overlying nerve compressions can change the natural history of the disease [73]. This is quite impressive in spite of a recent review article that does not even mention the role of surgery in diabetic neuropathy [74].

A study of the long-term results of carpal tunnel decompression reported on 60 patients, 10 of whom had diabetes. Decompression led to improvement in 86% of the patients overall (71% had marked improvement or complete recovery). Diabetes did not give a poor prognosis, but diabetic patients did have a slight trend toward less pain relief [75]. A recent study of outcomes of carpal tunnel release compared 22 patients who had diabetes with 25 non-diabetic patients. They found that a significant improvement in all of the parameters occurred in both groups after decompression of the median nerve at the carpal tunnel, but the magnitude of the improvement in the diabetics was not as great as the improvement in the non-diabetics [76]. A more recent study of the outcomes of carpal tunnel decompression in diabetics compared 24 patients who had diabetes with 72 non-diabetic patients and found that diabetes was not a risk factor for poor outcome; the diabetic patients had the same probability of positive surgical outcome. Improvement in subjective symptoms, measured with the Boston Questionnaire, was noted in 95.8% of diabetic patients at 6 months; objective improvement, measured by distal motor latency, was noted in 91.7% of diabetic patients at 6 months [77].

A study of cisplatin-induced neuropathy in Sprague-Dawley rats demonstrated that walking track abnormalities were prevented by early tarsal tunnel decompression. However, the decompressive surgery did not alter the walking track pattern if it was performed late, after neuropathy was established [57]. The results of this study showed that as it was developing, the cisplatin neuropathy could be reversed. Early monitoring of patients on cisplatin is critical in order to identify patients who might be treated with nerve decompressions.

Recent reports of thalidomide-induced neuropathy and symptomatic improvement following nerve decompression surgery have surfaced. (Michael Rose and A. Lee Dellon, personal communication, 2005). Additionally, peripheral nerve surgeons from various practices have reported the first nine surgically treated chemotherapy-induced neuropathy patients in *Plastic and Reconstructive Surgery* [58]. These patients suffered peripheral neuropathy from cisplatin, paclitaxel, and vincristine. All of these patients fit the World Health Organization's clinical definition of chemotherapy-induced neuropathy. Multiple nerves were decompressed in six of the nine patients; it was those six patients who were formally studied for outcome results. All six patients had pain relief ($P < .05$). In fact, three patients had a second limb and one patient had a third limb decompressed. Six out of six patients considered themselves to be functionally asymptomatic and had a preoperative neuropathy grade of 3 that declined to a neuropathy grade of 0.

Six out of six patients had some two-point discrimination improvement and four out of the six actually regained normal two-point discrimination in the limbs that had surgery. Most of the patients did have some type of nerve regeneration pain and continued on all of their preoperative medications for approximately 6 months before starting to taper medication. The paper noted that the electrophysiologic (EMG and nerve conduction) studies were not well tolerated by the patients. Electrophysiologic studies are difficult to use to assess chemotherapy-induced neuropathies, and it is important to rely on clinical examination [4]. The discussion stressed that the initial clinical experience of this group of surgeons relied on using the pressure specified sensory device, because it was non-invasive, well tolerated by the patients, and could easily be repeated and followed over time [58]. This study demonstrated findings in contradistinction to one of the major reviews of chemotherapy-induced peripheral neuropathy [4], which stated that there are no effective treatments to prevent or cure painful neuropathic symptoms caused by chemotherapy when it becomes disabling and severe. This retrospective study, in fact, showed that these patients did subjectively improve, and that this improvement most likely resulted from removal of the overlying nerve compressions at the usual sites of entrapment.

Cancer patients are now enjoying longer disease-free intervals because of the improvements in chemotherapy regimens As we strive to provide high quality of life for cancer patients, we should be acutely aware that there are surgical options for patients who fail medical treatment. The only published study to report decompression of peripheral nerves in chemotherapy-induced neuropathy in humans, evaluated only six patients, and so we eagerly await reports and published studies from other centers on their experiences with nerve decompression in patients with chemotherapy-induced neuropathy.

Acknowledgments

I thank Gracie Ink for assistance with the preparation of this manuscript.

References

[1] Visovsky C. Chemotherapy-induced peripheral neuropathy. Cancer Invest 2003;21(3): 439–51.
[2] Forman AD. Peripheral neuropathy and cancer. Curr Oncol Rep 2004;6(1):20–5.
[3] Ocean AJ, Vahdat LT. Chemotherapy-induced peripheral neuropathy: pathogenesis and emerging therapies. Support Care Cancer 2004;12(9):619–25.
[4] Quasthoff S, Hartung HP. Chemotherapy-induced peripheral neuropathy. J Neurol 2002; 249(1):9–17.
[5] Repetto L. Greater risks of chemotherapy toxicity in elderly patients with cancer. J Support Oncol 2003;1(4,Suppl 2):18–24.
[6] Weimer LH. Medication-induced peripheral neuropathy. Curr Neurol Neurosci Rep 2003; 3(1):86–92.

[7] Perkins BA, Olaleye D, Bril V. Carpal tunnel syndrome in patients with diabetic polyneuropathy. Diabetes Care 2002;25(3):565–9.

[8] Dellon AL. Measuring peripheral nerve function: electrodiagnostic versus neurosensory testing. Atlas Hand Clin 2005;10(1):1–31.

[9] Tanner KD, Levine JD, Topp KS. Microtubule disorientation and axonal swelling in unmyelinated sensory axons during vincristine-induced painful neuropathy in rat. J Comp Neurol 1998;395(4):481–92.

[10] Legha SS. Vincristine neurotoxicity. Pathophysiology and management. Med Toxicol 1986; 1(6):421–7.

[11] Peltier AC, Russell JW. Recent advances in drug-induced neuropathies. Curr Opin Neurol 2002;15(5):633–8.

[12] Kedar A, Cohen ME, Freeman AI. Peripheral neuropathy as a complication of cis-dichlorodiammineplatinum(II) treatment: a case report. Cancer Treat Rep 1978;62(5):819–21.

[13] Cersosimo RJ. Cisplatin neurotoxicity. Cancer Treat Rev 1989;16(4):195–211.

[14] Thompson SW, Davis LE, Kornfeld M, et al. Cisplatin neuropathy. Clinical, electrophysiologic, morphologic, and toxicologic studies. Cancer 1984;54(7):1269–75.

[15] Mollman JE. Cisplatin neurotoxicity. N Engl J Med 1990;322(2):126–7.

[16] Cavaletti G, Bogliun G, Marzorati L, et al. Early predictors of peripheral neurotoxicity in cisplatin and paclitaxel combination chemotherapy. Ann Oncol 2004;15(9):1439–42.

[17] Grothey A. Oxaliplatin-safety profile: neurotoxicity. Semin Oncol 2003;30(4,Suppl 15): 5–13.

[18] Cersosimo RJ. Oxaliplatin-associated neuropathy: a review. Ann Pharmacother 2005;39(1): 128–35.

[19] Cavaletti G, Tredici G, Braga M, et al. Experimental peripheral neuropathy induced in adult rats by repeated intraperitoneal administration of taxol. Exp Neurol 1995;133(1):64–72.

[20] Sahenk Z, Barohn R, New P, et al. Taxol neuropathy. Electrodiagnostic and sural nerve biopsy findings. Arch Neurol 1994;51(7):726–9.

[21] Rowinsky EK, Eisenhauer EA, Chaudhry V, et al. Clinical toxicities encountered with paclitaxel (Taxol). Semin Oncol 1993;20(4,Suppl 3):1–15.

[22] Pronk LC, Stoter G, Verweij J. Docetaxel (Taxotere): single agent activity, development of combination treatment and reducing side-effects. Cancer Treat Rev 1995;21(5):463–78.

[23] Hilkens PH, Verweij J, Stoter G, et al. Peripheral neurotoxicity induced by docetaxel. Neurology 1996;46(1):104–8.

[24] Verweij J, Clavel M, Chevalier B. Paclitaxel (Taxol) and docetaxel (Taxotere): not simply two of a kind. Ann Oncol 1994;5(6):495–505.

[25] Shapiro CL, Recht A. Side effects of adjuvant treatment of breast cancer. N Engl J Med 2001; 344(26):1997–2008.

[26] Chaudhry V, Eisenberger MA, Sinibaldi VJ, et al. A prospective study of suramin-induced peripheral neuropathy. Brain 1996;119(Pt 6):2039–52.

[27] Russell JW, Gill JS, Sorenson EJ, et al. Suramin-induced neuropathy in an animal model. J Neurol Sci 2001;192(1,2):71–80.

[28] Ghobrial IM, Rajkumar SV. Management of thalidomide toxicity. J Support Oncol 2003; 1(3):194–205.

[29] D'Amato RJ, Loughnan MS, Flynn E, et al. Thalidomide is an inhibitor of angiogenesis. Proc Natl Acad Sci USA 1994;91(9):4082–5.

[30] Raje N, Anderson K. Thalidomide–a revival story. N Engl J Med 1999;341(21):1606–9.

[31] Coleman M, Leonard J, Lyons L, et al. Treatment of Waldenstrom's macroglobulinemia with clarithromycin, low-dose thalidomide, and dexamethasone. Semin Oncol 2003;30(2): 270–4.

[32] Chaudhry V, Cornblath DR, Corse A, et al. Thalidomide-induced neuropathy. Neurology 2002;59(12):1872–5.

[33] Briani C, Zara G, Rondinone R, et al. Thalidomide neurotoxicity: prospective study in patients with lupus erythematosus. Neurology 2004;62(12):2288–90.

[34] Cavaletti G, Beronio A, Reni L, et al. Thalidomide sensory neurotoxicity: a clinical and neurophysiologic study. Neurology 2004;62(12):2291–3.

[35] Apfel SC, Zochodne DW. Thalidomide neuropathy: too much or too long? Neurology 2004; 62(12):2158–9.

[36] Dimopoulos MA, Eleutherakis-Papaiakovou V. Adverse effects of thalidomide administration in patients with neoplastic diseases. Am J Med 2004;117(7):508–15.

[37] Aghajanian C, Soignet S, Dizon DS, et al. A phase I trial of the novel proteasome inhibitor PS341 in advanced solid tumor malignancies. Clin Cancer Res 2002;8(8):2505–11.

[38] Maki RG, Kraft AS, Scheu K, et al. A multicenter Phase II study of bortezomib in recurrent or metastatic sarcomas. Cancer 2005;103(7):1431–8.

[39] Richardson PG, Barlogie B, Berenson J, et al. A phase 2 study of bortezomib in relapsed, refractory myeloma. N Engl J Med 2003;348(26):2609–17.

[40] Jagannath S, Barlogie B, Berenson J, et al. A phase 2 study of two doses of bortezomib in relapsed or refractory myeloma. Br J Haematol 2004;127(2):165–72.

[41] Goy A, Younes A, McLaughlin P, et al. Phase II study of proteasome inhibitor bortezomib in relapsed or refractory B-cell non-Hodgkin's lymphoma. J Clin Oncol 2005;23(4):667–75.

[42] Eng C, Kindler HL, Nattam S, et al. A phase II trial of the epothilone B analog, BMS-247550, in patients with previously treated advanced colorectal cancer. Ann Oncol 2004; 15(6):928–32.

[43] Low JA, Wedam SB, Lee JJ, et al. Phase II clinical trial of ixabepilone (BMS-247550), an epothilone B analog, in metastatic and locally advanced breast cancer. J Clin Oncol 2005; 23(12):2726–34.

[44] Galsky MD, Small EJ, Oh WK, et al. Multi-institutional randomized phase II trial of the epothilone B analog ixabepilone (BMS-247550) with or without estramustine phosphate in patients with progressive castrate metastatic prostate cancer. J Clin Oncol 2005;23(7): 1439–46.

[45] Chong PH, Boskovich A, Stevkovic N, et al. Statin-associated peripheral neuropathy: review of the literature. Pharmacotherapy 2004;24(9):1194–203.

[46] Bressler AM, Zimmer SM, Gilmore JL, et al. Peripheral neuropathy associated with prolonged use of linezolid. Lancet Infect Dis 2004;4(8):528–31.

[47] Cunha BA. Antibiotic side effects. Med Clin North Am 2001;85(1):149–85.

[48] Brew BJ. The peripheral nerve complications of human immunodeficiency virus (HIV) infection. Muscle Nerve 2003;28(5):542–52.

[49] Honnorat J, Cartalat-Carel S. Advances in paraneoplastic neurological syndromes. Curr Opin Oncol 2004;16(6):614–20.

[50] Altaha R, Abraham J. Paraneoplastic neurologic syndrome associated with occult breast cancer: a case report and review of literature. Breast J 2003;9(5):417–9.

[51] Rojas-Marcos I, Rousseau A, Keime-Guibert F, et al. Spectrum of paraneoplastic neurologic disorders in women with breast and gynecologic cancer. Medicine (Baltimore) 2003; 82(3):216–23.

[52] Koller H, Kieseier BC, Jander S, et al. Chronic inflammatory demyelinating polyneuropathy. N Engl J Med 2005;352(13):1343–56.

[53] Backonja M, Beydoun A, Edwards KR, et al. Gabapentin for the symptomatic treatment of painful neuropathy in patients with diabetes mellitus: a randomized controlled trial. JAMA 1998;280(21):1831–6.

[54] Beydoun A, Backonja MM. Mechanistic stratification of antineuralgic agents. J Pain Symptom Manage 2003;25(5 Suppl):S18–30.

[55] Wolfe GI, Trivedi JR. Painful peripheral neuropathy and its nonsurgical treatment. Muscle Nerve 2004;30(1):3–19.

[56] Gilron I, Bailey JM, Tu D, et al. Morphine, gabapentin, or their combination for neuropathic pain. N Engl J Med 2005;352(13):1324–34.

[57] Tassler P, Dellon AL, Lesser GJ, et al. Utility of decompressive surgery in the prophylaxis and treatment of cisplatin neuropathy in adult rats. J Reconstr Microsurg 2000;16(6):457–63.

[58] Dellon AL, Swier P, Maloney CT Jr, et al. Chemotherapy-induced neuropathy: treatment by decompression of peripheral nerves. Plast Reconstr Surg 2004;114(2):478–83.
[59] Dellon AL, Mackinnon SE, Seiler WA 4th. Susceptibility of the diabetic nerve to chronic compression. Ann Plast Surg 1988;20(2):117–9.
[60] Albers JW, Brown MB, Sima AA, et al. Frequency of median mononeuropathy in patients with mild diabetic neuropathy in the early diabetes intervention trial (EDIT). Muscle Nerve 1996;19(2):140–6.
[61] Dellon AL, Dellon ES, Seiler WA 4th. Effect of tarsal tunnel decompression in the strepto-zotocin-induced diabetic rat. Microsurgery 1994;15(4):265–8.
[62] Kale B, Yuksel F, Celikoz B, et al. Effect of various nerve decompression procedures on the functions of distal limbs in streptozotocin-induced diabetic rats: further optimism in diabetic neuropathy. Plast Reconstr Surg 2003;111(7):2265–72.
[63] Belgrade MJ, Lev BI. Diabetic neuropathy. Helping patients cope with their pain. Postgrad Med 1991;90(5):263–70.
[64] Vinik AI. Advances in diabetes for the millennium: new treatments for diabetic neuropa-thies. MedGenMed 2004;6(2):13.
[65] Dellon AL. Treatment of symptomatic diabetic neuropathy by surgical decompression of multiple peripheral nerves. Plast Reconstr Surg 1992;89(4):689–97 [discussion: 698–9].
[66] Wieman TJ, Patel VG. Treatment of hyperesthetic neuropathic pain in diabetics. Decom-pression of the tarsal tunnel. Ann Surg 1995;221(6):660–4 [discussion: 664–5].
[67] Aszmann OC, Kress KM, Dellon AL. Results of decompression of peripheral nerves in diabetics: a prospective, blinded study. Plast Reconstr Surg 2000;106(4):816–22.
[68] Caffee HH. Treatment of diabetic neuropathy by decompression of the posterior tibial nerve. Plast Reconstr Surg 2000;106(4):813–5.
[69] Tambwekar DS. Extended neurolysis of the posterior tibial nerve to improve sensation in diabetic neuropathic feet. Plast Reconstr Surg 2001;108(5):1452–3.
[70] Wood WA, Wood MA. Decompression of peripheral nerves for diabetic neuropathy in the lower extremity. J Foot Ankle Surg 2003;42(5):268–75.
[71] Biddinger KR, Amend KJ. The role of surgical decompression for diabetic neuropathy. Foot Ankle Clin 2004;9(2):239–54.
[72] Lee CH, Dellon AL. Prognostic ability of Tinel sign in determining outcome for decompres-sion surgery in diabetic and nondiabetic neuropathy. Ann Plast Surg 2004;53(6):523–7.
[73] Aszmann O, Tassler PL, Dellon AL. Changing the natural history of diabetic neuropathy: incidence of ulcer/amputation in the contralateral limb of patients with a unilateral nerve decompression procedure. Ann Plast Surg 2004;53(6):517–22.
[74] Singh N, Armstrong DG, Lipsky BA. Preventing foot ulcers in patients with diabetes. JAMA 2005;293(2):217–28.
[75] Haupt WF, Wintzer G, Schop A, et al. Long-term results of carpal tunnel decompression. Assessment of 60 cases. J Hand Surg [Br] 1993;18(4):471–4.
[76] Ozkul Y, Sabuncu T, Kocabey Y, et al. Outcomes of carpal tunnel release in diabetic and non-diabetic patients. Acta Neurol Scand 2002;106(3):168–72.
[77] Mondelli M, Padua L, Reale F, et al. Outcome of surgical release among diabetics with carpal tunnel syndrome. Arch Phys Med Rehabil 2004;85(1):7–13.

ELSEVIER
SAUNDERS

Clin Podiatr Med Surg
23 (2006) 651–666

CLINICS IN
PODIATRIC
MEDICINE AND
SURGERY

Physical Therapy Following Peripheral Nerve Surgeries

Tamara J. Bond, PT[a],*, Jim Lundy, DPT[b]

[a]Foot and Ankle Institute of Santa Monica, 2121 Wilshire Blvd, Suite 101,
Santa Monica, CA 90403, USA
[b]Athletic Physical Therapy, Los Angeles, CA, USA

Post-operative care of the surgical patient significantly contributes to the success of the surgical procedure. The goal of physical therapy is to return the patient to their pre-operative level of functioning or better by addressing the post-operative problems (Box 1).

Post-operative physical therapy is directed at reducing pain and inflammation, preventing or minimizing scar tissue, and returning the patient to full function. An individualized and well-planned therapeutic exercise program is an integral part of the post-operative care. Manual therapy techniques are utilized to break up scar tissue and reduce joint stiffness. Pain and inflammation can be addressed by modalities such as ultrasound, laser, and electrical stimulation in addition to cryotherapy.

Patient self-involvement is paramount for success at all stages in rehabilitation. Patients must be strongly advised that their participation will advance the healing process and absence of involvement may delay progress.

Physical therapy is usually divided up into three stages and each stage has specific impairments and treatment goals to address (Table 1). The three stages can vary in length, which is based upon an individual patients' condition.

Stage 1

The patient is referred to physical therapy when the surgeon has deemed gentle movement to be appropriate for their level of healing. Typically the first 2 weeks of physical therapy will involve active and active-assisted range of motion (ROM) exercises, education about pain management and the healing process, gentle joint mobilizations to improve range of motion

---

* Corresponding author.
E-mail address: tamara@athleticpt.com (T.J. Bond).

0891-8422/06/$ - see front matter © 2006 Elsevier Inc. All rights reserved.
doi:10.1016/j.cpm.2006.04.006
podiatric.theclinics.com

Box 1. Post-operative problems

Pain secondary to disruption of soft tissue
Edema
Circulatory complications
Joint stiffness/limitation of motion secondary to soft tissue injury
    and post-operative immobilization
Muscle atrophy as a result of immobilization
Loss of strength for functional activities
Limitation of weight bearing
Potential loss of strength and mobility in uninvolved joints

---

and reduce pain, gentle soft tissue massage to reduce swelling, modalities to address pain and inflammation, and light resisted exercises to increase strength.

Stage 2

During the second stage, treatments for ROM and strength will be advanced as the patient tolerates more weight-bearing resistive devices and closed kinetic chain exercises. More aggressive joint mobilization will be incorporated, as well as scar mobilization, in addition to laser and ultrasound therapy to improve scar tissue. Also in this stage, gait training will address any gait abnormalities and deficits developed pre- or post-surgery. Initial introduction to balance training will be incorporated to develop appropriate neuromuscular response throughout the lower kinetic chain. Electrical stimulation and ice may be applied at the end of each treatment to negate any edema, which may have ensued during treatment.

Table 1
Stages and goals of post-operative rehabilitation

Rehabilitation stage	Time frame	Goal of stage
Stage 1	3–5 weeks post-op	↓ Edema
		↓ Pain
		↑ ROM
Stage 2	5–7 weeks post-op	↑ Strength
		↑ ROM
		Normalize gait
		Begin balance training
Stage 3	7–10 weeks post-op	↑ Balance/proprioception
		↑ Maximize strength/ROM
		Full functional return

Abbreviation: ROM, range of motion.

Stage 3

During the third and final stage of rehabilitation, closed kinetic chain exercises will become more advanced to challenge the patient's balance and proprioception. Strength, endurance and flexibility exercises will continue to progress until the operated side is within normal limits. The addition of functional exercises will allow for full return to activities of daily life and athletic activities. Lastly, therapeutic modalities and cryotherapy may continue to be applied with discretion to address any lasting pain or inflammation at the surgical site.

Range of motion exercises

The appropriate time to begin physical therapy is often questioned. The effects of motion on nerve repair have not been very well studied. In current practices, surgeons generally immobilize the surrounding joints for 2–6 weeks after nerve repair.

Animal studies with median and ulnar nerve transection and repair indicate that early mobilization impedes nerve regeneration by increasing scar formation and delaying revascularization [1]. In the study group that was immobilized, revascularization crossed the neurorrhaphy in 3 weeks; however, within the mobilized group, a persistent "hypovascular zone" was present at the nerve repair site for up to 6 weeks. In rat sciatic nerve repair, range of motion impedes the functional nerve recovery by decreasing endoneural collagenization and decreasing angiogenesis [2]. Other animal studies also confirm the deleterious effects of early exercise on the healing of peripheral nerves in rats, but these studies involved high intensity exercises and negative reinforcements [3–7].

The application of passive motion on surgical repairs is controversial. In rabbit popliteal nerve transection and repair, continuous early passive motion sustained fewer and less dense adhesions, but showed slightly slower nerve conduction and less myelinated fiber regeneration [8]. Investigators concluded that the operated limb does not have to be immobilized in order for nerve regeneration to take place.

Exercises should be progressed gradually during the early post-operative period, because soft tissues, which were disrupted during surgery, will be inflamed. It is important to continually note the level of swelling and pain; if there is a marked increase, exercises should be temporarily discontinued or reduced in intensity.

After immobilization, there will be loss of range of motion, muscle atrophy, and pain. In order to minimize trauma to the weakened tissues, activities should be initiated carefully. Recovery may be delayed when exercises or functional activity progress too quickly because they may perpetuate the inflammatory response [9,10].

Begin with active-assisted and active joint motion to improve and maintain the length and mobility of muscle and soft tissue. When pain is felt only at the end-range of the available range of motion, the therapist applies manual passive stretches to elongate tissue past their resting length. A slow maintained stretch is indicated, because it is less likely to facilitate the stretch reflex and increase tension in the muscle being lengthened. The stretch is usually applied for 15–30 seconds. Hallum and Mederios [11] found that a 15-second stretch was just as effective as a 45-second or 2-minute stretch. The gains achieved in range of motion are the result of elastic changes in actin-myosin overlap [12]. The physical therapist may use a technique called active inhibition to reflexively relax the muscle before elongation. Either a contract-relax technique or a contraction of the antagonistic muscle is used to inhibit the tight muscle and facilitate further stretch into the end range [13].

Scar tissue mobilization

The treatment goal is the formation of a strong, mobile scar and complete and painless restoration of function. An inelastic scar will lead to decreased range of motion or pain when placed on a stretch. It is essential to mobilize the scar tissue to regain painless movement. Adhesions of the fascia, skin, or other soft tissue such as the ligaments will restrict joint motion and should be mobilized. Stretching techniques should be specific to the area. Cross-fiber massage or transverse friction massage is advocated to keep the developing scar mobile [14,15]. Scar tissue mobilization should begin once complete closure of the wound has occurred. Lee et al and Millesi report that scar tissue impedes axonal sprouting and thus nerve regeneration [16,17].

Manual therapy

When needed, manual therapy mobilizations are performed to prevent scar tissue adhesions from restricting joint movement. To decrease post-surgical stiffness and pain, joint mobilizations are manual techniques used to restore joint dysfunction [18]. Local massage may benefit circulation to decrease swelling and pain.

Because of the post-surgical immobilization period, specific joint mobilizations are indicated. Following neuroma resection or decompression, flexion of the adjacent metatarsal phalangeal joints may be restricted. Traction, plantar glides, and flexion mobilizations of the metatarsal phalangeal joints are performed as well as plantar and dorsal glides of the adjacent metatarsals. When the peroneal nerve has been released, anterior-lateral and posterior-medial glides of the fibular head on the proximal tibia are performed to address adhesions of the superior tibio-fibular joint. Rarely are joint mobilizations required when tarsal tunnel is released because of the common pre-existing ankle or foot laxity present. When ankle dorsi-flexion is limited, posterior glide of the talus on the tibia is performed. Other less common joint mobilizations may be necessary, however, the reader is referred to other sources [19,20].

Strengthening and endurance exercises

Post-operative disuse and immobilization will result in muscle weakness. Strength gains are made as a result of hypertrophy of muscle fiber and increased recruitment of motor units in the muscle [21,22]. Resistance exercises are an integral part of post-operative physical therapy.

Exercise training improves the return of sensomotoric function in the case of a crushed peripheral nerve [23]. Beneficial effects were seen in the early phase of recovery and persisted into the late phase. Research suggests that the speed of axonal sprouting increases with exercise training [24].

Manual resisted exercises, in which the therapist applies resistance, are indicated in the early stages of rehabilitation. Manual resistance allows for mild to moderate amounts of resistance and carefully controlled motion. Isometric resistance may also be used during early strengthening. Isotonic concentric and eccentric resistance exercises are progressed with the use of external equipment by moving from open to closed kinetic chain exercises, and by increasing the tension of elastic tubing, weights, or pulleys.

Recent studies [25,26] purport that the mechanical efficiency of the neuromuscular system is improved with strength training. Strength training improves intermuscular coordination by a more consistent recruitment of motor units. Strength gains can also be achieved while re-training balance [27,28].

Endurance is gained by performing many repetitions against mild resistance [29]. Muscular endurance has also been shown to increase with an exercise program designed to increase strength [30].

Balance, proprioception, and sensorimotor training

A crucial component of the final rehabilitation phase involves balance activities that challenge the sensorimotor system. Activities progress in a gradual manner, and safety (fall prevention) is a constant concern. Balance exercises begin with double-leg balance, feet in various positions, and eyes open. Perturbations, upper-extremity reaching, and cervical/lumbar spinal movements are added challenges at this stage (Fig. 1). Balancing on a single leg or with eyes closed advances the exercises (Fig. 2).

The sensorimotor component of balance re-training involves maintaining postural stability while standing on unstable surfaces: wobble boards (Fig. 3), spinning tops (Fig. 4), soft mats, or a stabilometer training device. This training improves overall lower extremity muscular control, which ultimately maximizes dynamic joint stability in the foot and ankle complex. The efficiency of activating high muscular force in short time periods

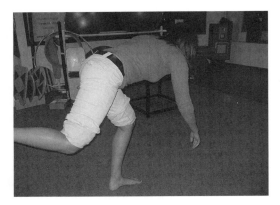

Fig. 1. Balance activity with forward reaching.

appears to be critical in creating this stability. This is especially important in injury related situations [31–33].

Gait training

An assistive device should be used for ambulation until strength of the lower extremity has improved to a grade of Fair (3/5) with strength testing as per Kendall et al [34].

Neurological changes occur in the first 6 weeks of a rehabilitation program and early therapy should focus on coordinated movement and gait patterns to avoid long term compensations [34].

After immobilization, several common gait corrections are usually required: equalizing stride length and the time spent on each leg, improving heel-toe gait pattern and push-off, improving gluteus medius strength to address hip drop, and equalizing arm swing.

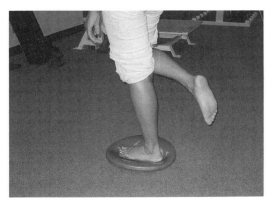

Fig. 2. Unilateral balance on unstable surface.

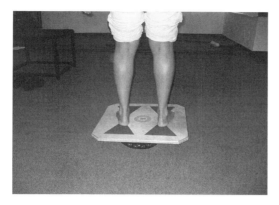

Fig. 3. Balance on wobble board.

Ultrasound

Pulsed (non-thermal) ultrasound may be used initially to reduce post-operative pain and inflammation when the incision is fully closed. Later, ultrasound can be set to a continuous mode to heat the scar before cross-fiber massage. This also increases blood flow, reduces pain and muscle spasm, and increases tissue extensibility [35].

Ultrasound can be used to improve nerve regeneration after injury, compression, or outright crush of the peripheral nerve. Although ultrasound has been used to treat a variety of disorders in the orthopedic realm, nerve regeneration in peripheral nerves is a new application. In post-surgical situations where there may be nerve compression, ultrasound provides an additional tool to assist with regeneration. Research to date has been focused on animal subjects; there has been minimal research on nerve regeneration in human subjects.

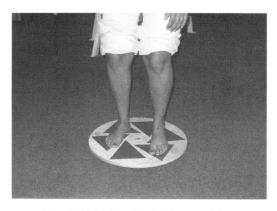

Fig. 4. Multi-directional balance activity.

The research in pulsed altrasound has investigated both complete nerve lesions as well as crush injuries. In the case of tenotomy of the sciatic nerve, research indicates that there are significant gains in the number of the larger A and B type fibers as well as gains in sheath thickness [36]. Morphological investigations have shown that Schwann cells appear more to be metabolically active compared with controls. In short term application, ultrasound appears to positively affect nerves that are myelinated.

The positive influence of pulsed ultrasound on Schwann cells is further supported in tenotomy and conduit situations [37]. In surgical conduits between two portions of an excised and removed nerve segment, especially those packed with Schwann cells, ultrasound demonstrated a significant increase in the number and area of myelinated axons.

In more crush type injuries, improved functional return and increased nerve fiber density in the segments distal to the injury were noted [38]. It was suggested that nerve sprouting and increased stimulation of Schwann cells could explain the improved nerve fiber density in animals treated with pulsed ultrasound. In other crush situations, functional return has been noted starting 14 days after injury using short duration continuous wave ultrasound [39].

There has been confusion about the intensity of ultrasound applications. When edema is present in compression situations, higher intensities of continuous ultrasound (1.5 W/cm^2) demonstrated improved compound muscle action potentials (CMAP) in the rabbit median nerve, compared with lower power levels (0.2 W/cm^2) [40]. In the rat tibial nerve, lower intensities of continuous wave (0.5 W/cm^2) improve nerve conduction velocity and CMAP compared with higher intensities (1.0 W/cm^2) [41]. The treatment times between studies varied between rat (1 min, 3 times per week) and rabbit (5 min, 5 times per week) nerves. Because these were acute compressions and ultrasound was applied continuously, the primary treatment effect appears to be thermal. In healthy human subjects, the thermal effects on subcutaneous tissue appear to alter motor and sensory nerve latencies compared with nonthermal and mechanical effects [42]. Although acute compressions are not seen frequently in the lower extremity, long-term compressions of lower extremity nerves will most likely necessitate surgical intervention. Because post-surgical edema may be surrounding nerves, ultrasound may alleviate edema to further assist with nerve conduction.

In the clinic setting, pulsed ultrasound is used when significant edema is present. As edema resolves, continuous ultrasound is applied directly over the nerve and incision site (Fig. 5).

Low level laser therapy

Low level laser therapy (LLLT), laser therapy, or simply phototherapy is the application of light waves to produce a biological effect on the living tissue. Although this modality has a long history and has been used in other

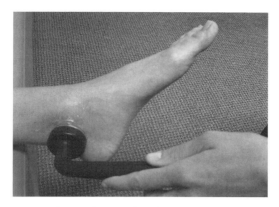

Fig. 5. Ultrasound to the tarsal tunnel.

countries, it was approved within the United States for pain management in 2002. Subsequently, many medical professionals have shown increased interest in this modality [43,44]. Low level lasers in the red and infrared light spectrum use wavelengths between 540 nm and 840 nm and power outputs between 5 mW and 500 mW. The laser intensities are low enough to not produce thermal effects in the treated area, and are not perceptible to sensation.

Although previous research has focused on a variety of orthopedic and non-orthopedic disorders such as chronic pain [45,46], tendonitis [47–49], myofascial pain [50–53], osteoarthritis [54–56], and headaches [57], current research in nerve disorders has demonstrated both sensory and motor nerve benefits. Within human peripheral nerve compression syndromes, especially in the carpal tunnel region, lasers have demonstrated decreased sensory nerve conduction latencies and improved pain relief with three treatments per week for 3–4 weeks [58]. Additionally, many clinical tests that were initially positive, reverted to negative post treatment. Pain relief and multiple sensory nerve deficits have improved with the use of LLLT in human facial surgery [59]. Treatments up to 30 minutes for 21 days demonstrated significantly increased positive somatosensory evoked response, increased number of axons, and increased number of large-diameter axons in the irradiated sciatic nerve of rats compared with controls [60].

Most research has used animal studies although there have been a few human studies. The initial use of LLLT on peripheral nerve regeneration used a helium-neon laser and irradiated the crushed sciatic nerve for 7 minutes per day for 21 days [61]. CMAP of the crushed nerve dropped to 60% of pre-crush measurements (40% controls) initially after injury and increased to higher levels at 3 weeks and 1 year later. Higher levels of CMAP in peripheral nerves were noted post-injury with direct irradiation to the spinal cord and no peripheral application [62]. Thus, both peripheral and central stimulation appear to improve CMAP in peripheral nerves. The significant difference in CMAP between the irradiated and non-irradiated nerve indicates LLLT enhances peripheral nerve regeneration.

Another benefit of LLLT as a post-surgery rehabilitation modality is pain inhibition or alleviation. Animal studies indicate that painful chemical and mechanical stimuli on nerves can be abated with low level laser treatment. Irradiation to unmyelinated sensory A delta fibers consistently suppressed nerve impulse conduction in rats [63–65] and rabbits [66]. This pain relieving analgesia may be an additional adjunct to current treatment.

LLLT has several mechanisms by which it may assist and encourage peripheral nerve regeneration. First, laser therapy has an effect on the growth cone or leading edge of a nerve cell. In fact, the irradiation can lead the nerve cell to encourage development toward the irradiated area [67]. Second, laser therapy at a cellular level will increase mitochondria activity, oxidation, and subsequent cellular activity (R. Martin, PhD, personal communication, June, 2005). Third, laser irradiation to an injured nerve directly effects and increases nerve sprouting because of cellular respiratory activation by cytochromes and ATP production. Finally, in addition to cellular stimulation, LLLT has been shown to increase the number of growth present antibody neurons (growth-associated protein-43) in animals within 3 weeks post crush injury, significantly more than non-irradiated nerves [68]. Therefore, low level laser therapy has multiple mechanisms of action that regenerate peripheral nerve lesions.

From a clinical perspective, application of LLLT should be addressed at the site of nerve lesion (Fig. 6). The research on nerve regeneration was applied immediately after nerve resection and repair, and LLLT should be applied to the nerve as soon as feasible post surgery.

Electrical stimulation

Although much research exists regarding other modalities, the use of electrical stimulation appears most logical as an initial treatment modality for

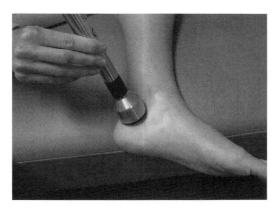

Fig. 6. Low level LASER to the tarsal tunnel.

peripheral nerve injuries. Because electrical stimulation exerts its action on the nerve similar to its in vivo mechanism, it is naturally a viable adjunct to post-surgical rehabilitation. Research in this area has existed for many years but only recently has elucidated possible mechanisms for its effect.

Previous animal research has investigated electrical stimulation on peripheral motor and sensory nerves. Within crushed nerve research, stimulation of between 5 minutes and 1 hour, directly on the crushed rat nerve, significantly increased speed of regeneration but not number of axons regenerating [69]. Although longer duration stimulation improved motor function [70], the most critical time to induce regeneration is immediately post injury (no delay). In addition to increased functional return, histological studies indicate that stimulation results in a higher density of small diameter fibers and increased number and diameter of intraneural blood vessels [71].

There is supportive evidence for electrical stimulation in animal studies. Direct electrical stimulation in transected and repaired rat sciatic and femoral nerves for 2 weeks resulted in regeneration of motor axons within 3 weeks, versus 8–10 weeks without stimulation [72,73]. Surgically repaired sensory nerve regeneration also improves with electrical stimulation [74]. This effect was also produced with minimal stimulation (1 hr, 20 Hz) primarily at the nerve stump and not on the nerve distally. Other research indicates electrical stimulation significantly enhances the growth of new motor neurons during 1–2 weeks post repair without increasing the speed of axon growth [75]. The nerve regeneration speed (distance of growth per day) is minimally different between stimulation and control subjects; stimulation simply increases the number of new motor axons developed compared with controls. Stimulating the nerve before crush injury does not enhance post-injury regeneration. Thus, stimulation in absence of axonal injury does not enhance future growth of the motor neuron.

Electrical stimulation has also been found to affect muscle distal to a crush injury. Daily stimulation in denervated rat muscles resulted in less muscle loss, increased cross-sectional area, and increased contractile ability of the muscle [76,77]. Stimulation was applied between 2 months and 9 months post injury, although significant differences were unable to be assessed after 2 months in either study. However, as noted in other post injury research, electrical stimulation was most effective within 4 weeks of injury.

Although electrical stimulation improves motor and sensory regeneration post transection or crush injury, the mechanism for action is unclear. The cell body of the axon appears to be the primary site for activation of peripheral nerve regeneration in crush injuries. Neurotrophic factors, such as brain-derived neurotrophic factor (BDNF) and tyrosine receptor kinase B (trkB), and muscle derived factors, such as MDP77 [78], may contribute to axonal regeneration. The most research revolves around BDNF and trkB receptors in the motor neuron, which upon direct stimulation, have increased upregulation and acceleration in expression [79,80]. These effects are also correlated with peripheral motor axonal regeneration.

From the research, the clinical application of transcutaneous electrical stimulation should be instituted close to the nerve injury and with a minimal delay post surgery. The electrical stimulation electrodes can be place along the nerve path and distally on the muscle to be stimulated. Active motion with the stimulation would be encouraged unless wound issues preclude mobility.

Phonophoresis and iontophoresis

When post-operative complications such as a stump neuroma, neuritis, or excessive local swelling are present, iontophoresis or phonophoresis may be used. Iontophoresis is used to deliver a dexamethasone sodium phosphate to locally reduce inflammation and pain [81]. When topical medication is indicated, ultrasound can be used to increase the transdermal delivery of the medication [82]. Phonophoresis uses ultrasound to drive topical medications, such as corticosteroid or non-steroidal anti-inflammatory medications, into the tissue.

Summary

The goals of physical therapy in the post-operative period are to reduce pain and swelling, accelerate the healing process, prevent scar tissue from forming, and return the patient to full functional recovery.

Post-operative care of the surgical patient significantly contributes to the success of the surgical procedure. An individualized and well-planned therapeutic exercise program is an integral part of the post-operative care.

References

[1] Lee WP, Constantinescu MA, Butler PE. Effect of early mobilization on healing of nerve repair: histologic observations in a canine model. Plast Reconstr Surg 1999;104:1718–25.
[2] Schmidhammer R, Zandieh S, Hopf R, et al. Alleviated tension at the repair site enhances functional regeneration: the effect of full range of motion mobilization on the regeneration of peripheral nerves–histological, electrophysiologic, and functional results in a rat model. J Trauma 2004;56:571–84.
[3] Herbison GJ, Jaweed MM, Ditunno JF, et al. Effect of over-work during reinnervation of rat muscle. Exp Neurol 1973;41:1–14.
[4] Herbison GJ, Jaweed MM, Ditunno JF. Effect of swimming on reinnervation of rat skeletal muscle. J Neurol Neurosurg Psychiatry 1974;37:1247–51.
[5] Herbison GJ, Jaweed MM, Ditunno JF. Effect of activity and inactivity on reinnervating rat skeletal muscle contractility. Exp Neurol 1980;70:498–506.
[6] Herbison GJ, Jaweed MM, Ditunno JF. Histochemical fiber type alterations secondary to exercise training of reinnervating adult rat muscle. Arch Phys Med Rehabil 1980;61:355–7.
[7] Gutmann E, Jakoubek B. Effect of increased motor activity on regeneration of the peripheral nerve in young rats. Physiol Bohemoslov 1963;12:463–8.

[8] Kim HKW, Kerr RG, Turley CB, et al. The effects of post-operative continuous passive motion on peripheral nerve repair and regeneration. An experimental investigation in rabbits. J Hand Surg 1998;23B(5):594–7.

[9] Wilhelm DL. Inflammation and healing. In: Anderson WAD, editor. Pathology. St. Louis (MO): CV Mosby; 1971.

[10] Zohn D, Mennell J. Musculoskeletal pain: principles of physical therapy diagnosis and physical treatment. Boston: Little, Brown & Company; 1976.

[11] Hallum A, Medeiros JM. Effect of duration of passive stretch on hip abduction range of motion. J Orthop Sports Phys Ther 1987;18:409.

[12] Griffiths PJ, Goth K, Kuhn HJ, et al. Cross bridge slippage in skinned frog muscle fibers. Biophys Struct Mech 1980;7:107.

[13] Condon SN, Hutton RS. Soleus muscle electromyographic activity and ankle dorsi flexion range of motion during four stretching procedures. Phys Ther 1987;67:24.

[14] Chamberlain G. Cyriax's friction massage: a review. JOSPT 1982;4:16.

[15] Cyriax J. Textbook of orthopedic medicine, vol 1. Diagnosis of soft tissue lesions. 8th edition. London: Bailliere and Tindall; 1982.

[16] Lee AWP, Constantinescu MA, Butler PEM. Effect of early mobilization on healing of nerve repair: histologic observations in a canine model. Plas Recon Surg 1999;104(6):1718–25.

[17] Millesi H. Peripheral nerve repair: terminology, questions, and facts. J Reconstr Microsurg 1985;2:21.

[18] Cyriax J, Cyriax P. Cyriax's Illustrated Manual of Orthopedic Medicine. 2nd edition. Oxford: Butterworth Heinemann; 1996.

[19] Wadsworth CT. Manual examination and treatment of the spine and extremities. Baltimore (MD): Williams and Wilkins; 1988.

[20] Maitland GD. Vertebral manipulation. 5th edition. London: Butterworth Heinemann; 1986.

[21] Lehmkuhl LD, Smith LK. Brunnstrom's clinical kinesiology. 4th edition. Philadelphia: FA Davis; 1983.

[22] Wolf SL. The morphological and functional basis of therapeutic exercise. In: Basmajian JV, editor. Therapeutic exercise. 3rd edition. Baltimore: Williams and Wilkins; 1978.

[23] Van Meeteren NLU, Brakkee JH, Hamers FPT, et al. Exercise training improves functional recovery and motor conduction velocity after sciatic nerve crush lesion in the rat. Arch Phys Med Rehabil 1997;78:70–7.

[24] Vecchi G. Sulla rigenerazione del nervo sciatico in animali constretti alla corsa. Arch Sci Med (Torino) 1929;53:778–83.

[25] Bruhn S, Kullmann N, Gollhofer A. The effects of a sensorimotor training and a strength training on postural stabilization, maximum isometric contraction and jump performance. Int J Sports Med 2004;25:56–60.

[26] Carroll TJ, Barry B, Riek S, et al. Resistance training enhances the stability of the sensorimotor coordination. Proc R Soc Lond B Biol Sci 2001;268:221–7.

[27] Gruber M, Gollhofer A. Impact of sensorimotor training on the rate of force development and neural activation. Eur J Appl Physiol 2004;92:98–105.

[28] Heitkamp HC, Horstmann T, Mayer F, et al. Gain in strength and muscular balance after balance training. Int J Sports Med 2001;22:285–90.

[29] Darling RC. Exercise. In: Downey JA, Darling RC, editors. The physiological basis of rehabilitative medicine. Philadelphia: WB Saunders; 1971.

[30] DeLateur BJ. Therapeutic exercise to develop strength and endurance. In: Kottle FJ, Stillwell GK, Lehmann JF, editors. Krusen's handbook of physical medicine and rehabilitation. 3rd edition. Philadelphia: WB Saunders; 1982.

[31] Alt W, Lohrer H, Gollhofer A. Functional properties of adhesive ankle taping: neuromuscular and mechanical effects before and after exercise. Foot Ankle Int 1999;20:238–45.

[32] Bloem BR, Allum JH, Carpenter MG, et al. Is lower leg proprioception essential for triggering human automatic postural responses? Exp Brain Res 2000;130:375–91.

[33] Konradsen L, Olesen S, Hansen HM. Ankle sensorimotor control and eversion strength after acute ankle inversion injuries. Am J Sports Med 1998;26:72–7.

[34] Kendall FP, McCreary EK, Provance PG. Muscle testing and function. 3rd edition. Williams & Wilkins USA; 1996.

[35] Speed CA. Therapeutic ultrasound in soft tissue lesions. Rheumatology (Oxford) 2001;40: 1331–6.

[36] Crisci AR, Ferreira AL. Low-intensity pulsed ultrasound accelerates the regeneration of the sciatic nerve after neurotomy in rats. Ultrasound Med Biol 2002;28:1335–41.

[37] Chang CJ, Hsu SH. The effects of low-intensity ultrasound on peripheral nerve regeneration in poly (DL-lactic acid-co-glycolic acid) conduits seeded with schwann cells. Ultrasound Med Biol 2004;30:1079–84.

[38] Monte Raso VV, Barbieri CH, Mazzer N, et al. Can therapeutic ultrasound influence the regeneration of peripheral nerves? J Neurosci Meth 2005;142:185–92.

[39] Mourad PD, Lazar DA, Curro FP, et al. Ultrasound accelerated functional recover after peripheral nerve damage. Neurosurg 2001;48:1136–41.

[40] Paik NJ, Cho SH, Han TR. Ultrasound therapy facilitates the recovery of acute pressure-induced conduction block of the median nerve in rabbits. Muscle Nerve 2002;26:356–61.

[41] Hong CZ, Liu HH, Yu U. Ultrasound thermotherapy effect on the recovery of nerve conduction in experimental compression neuropathy. Arch Phys Med Rehabil 1988;69:410–4.

[42] Moore JH, Gieck JH, Saliba EN, et al. The biophysical effects of ultrasound on median nerve distal latencies. Electromyogr Clin Neurophysiol 2000;40:169–80.

[43] Gigo-Benato D, Geuna S, Rochkind S. Phototherapy for enhancing peripheral nerve repair: a review of the literature. Musc Nerv 2005;31:694–701.

[44] Anders JJ, Geuna S, Rochkind S. Phototherapy promotes regeneration and functional recovery of injured peripheral nerve. Neurol Res 2004;26:233–9.

[45] Chow R, Barnsley L, Heller G, et al. Efficacy of 300 mW, 830 nm laser in the treatment of chronic pain: a survey in a general practice setting. J Musculoskeletal Pain 2003;11:13–21.

[46] Fukuuchi A, Suzuki H, Inoue K. A double-blind trial of low reactive-level laser therapy in the treatment of chronic pain. Laser Ther 1998;10:59–64.

[47] Bjordal JM, Couppe C, Ljunggren E. Low level laser therapy for tendinopathy. Evidence of a dose-response pattern. Phys Ther Rev 2001;6:91–9.

[48] Logdberg-Andersson M, Mutzell S, Hazel A. Low level laser therapy (lllt) of tendonitis and myofascial pains: a randomized, double-blind controlled study. Laser Ther 1997;9:79–86.

[49] Simunovic S, Trobonjaca T, Trobonjaca Z. Treatment of medial and lateral epicondylitis-tennis and golfer's elbow-with low level laser therapy: a multicenter double blind, placebo-controlled clinical study on 324 patients. J Clin Laser Med Surg 1998;16:145–51.

[50] Laasko EL, Richardson C, Cramond T. Pain scores and side effects in response to low level laser therapy (lllt) for myofascial trigger points. Laser Ther 1997;9:67–72.

[51] Gur A, Karakoe M, Nas K, et al. Efficacy of low power laser therapy in fibromyalgia: a single-blind, placebo-controlled trial. Laser Med Sci 2002;17:57–61.

[52] Hakguder A, Birtane M, Gurcan S, et al. Efficacy of low level laser therapy in myofascial pain syndrome: an algometric and thermographic evaluation. Lasers Surg Med 2003;33: 339–43.

[53] Simunovic Z. LLLT with trigger points technique: a clinical study on 243 patients. J Clin Laser Med Surg 1996;14:163–7.

[54] Stelian J, Gil I, Habot B, et al. Improvement of pain and disability in elderly patients with degenerative osteoarthritis of the knee treated with narrow-band light therapy. J Am Geriatr Soc 1992;40:23–6.

[55] Oezdemir F, Birtane M, Kokion S. The clinical efficacy of low-power laser therapy on pain and function in cervical osteoarthritis. Clin Rheumatol 2001;20:181–4.

[56] Trelles MA, Riqau J, Sala P, et al. Infrared diode laser in low reactive-level laser therapy (lllt) for knee osteoarthritis. Laser Ther 1991;3:149–53.

[57] Allais G, De Lorenzo C, Quirico PE, et al. Non-pharmacological approaches to chronic headaches: transcutaneous electrical nerve stimulation, laser therapy, and acupuncture in transformed migraine treatment. Neurol Sci 2003;24(Suppl 2):S138–42.
[58] Naeser MA, Hahn KAK, Lieberman BE, et al. Carpal tunnel syndrome pain treated with low-level laser and microamperes transcutaneous electric nerve stimulation: a controlled study. Arch Phys Med Rehabil 2002;83:978–88.
[59] Miloro M, Repasky M. Low-level laser effect on neurosensory recovery after sagittal ramus osteotomy. Oral Surg Oral Med Oral Pathol Oral Radiol Endod 2000;89:12–8.
[60] Shamir MH, Rochkind S, Sandbank J, et al. Double-blind randomized study evaluating regeneration of the rat transected sciatic nerve after suturing and post-operative low-power laser treatment. J Reconstr Microsurg 2001;17:133–7.
[61] Rochkind S, Rousso M, Nissan M, et al. Systemic effects of low-power laser irradiation on the peripheral and central nervous system, cutaneous wounds, and burns. Laser Surg Med 1989;9:174–82.
[62] Rochkind S, Nissan M, Alon M, et al. Effects of laser irradiation on the spinal cord for the regeneration of crushed peripheral nerve in rats. Las Surg Med 2001;28:216–9.
[63] Tsuchiya K, Kawatani M, Takeshige C, et al. Laser irradiation abates neuronal responses to nociceptive stimulation of rat-paw skin. Brain Res Bull 1994;34:369–74.
[64] Wedlock PM, Shepard RA. Cranial irradiation with GaAlAs laser leads to naloxone reversible analgesia in rats. Psychol Rep 1996;78:727–31.
[65] Sato T, Kawatani M, Takeshige C, et al. Ga-Al-As laser irradiation inhibits neuronal activity associated with inflammation. Acupunct Electrother Res 1994;19:141–51.
[66] Kasai S, Kono T, Sakamoto T, et al. Effects of low-power laser irradiation on multiple unit discharges induced by noxious stimuli in the anesthetized rabbit. J Clin Laser Med Surg 1994;12:221–4.
[67] Ehrlicher A, Betz T, Stuhrmann B, et al. Guiding neuronal growth with light. Proc Natl Acad Sci USA 2002;99:16024–8.
[68] Shin DH, Lee E, Hyun JK, et al. Growth-associated protein-43 is elevated in the injured rat sciatic nerve after low power laser irradiation. Neurosci Lett 2003;344:71–4.
[69] Pockett S, Gavin RM. Acceleration of peripheral nerve regeneration after crush injury in rat. Neurosci Lett 1985;59:221–4.
[70] Nix WA, Hopf HC. Electrical stimulation of regenerating nerve and its effect on motor recovery. Brain Res 1983;272:21–5.
[71] Mendonca AC, Barbieri CH, Mazzer N. Directly applied low intensity direct electric current enhances peripheral nerve regeneration in rats. J Neurosci Methods 2003;129:183–90.
[72] Al-Majed AA, Neumann CM, Brushart TM, et al. Brief electrical stimulation promotes the speed and accuracy of motor axonal regeneration. J Neurosci 2000;20:2602–8.
[73] Gordon T, Sulaiman O, Boyd JG. Experimental strategies to promote functional recovery after peripheral nerve injuries. J Peripher Nerv Syst 2003;8:236–50.
[74] Brushart TM, Jari R, Verge V, et al. Electrical stimulation restores the specificity of sensory axon regeneration. Exp Neurol 2005;194:221–9.
[75] Brushart TM, Hoffman PN, Royall RM, et al. Electrical stimulation promotes motorneuron regeneration without increasing its speed or conditioning the neuron. J Neurosci 2002;22:6631–8.
[76] Cole BG, Gardiner PF. Does electrical stimulation of denervated muscle, continued after reinnervation, influence recovery of contractile function? Exp Neurol 1984;85:52–62.
[77] Hennig R, Lomo T. Effects of chronic stimulation on the size and speed of long-term denervated and innervated rat fast and slow skeletal muscles. Acta Physiol Scand 1987;130:115–31.
[78] Itoh S, Uyeda A, Hukuoka Y, et al. Muscle-specific protein MDP77 specifically promotes motor nerve regeneration in rats. Neurosci Lett 2004;360:175–7.

[79] Al-Majed AA, Brushart TM, Gordon T. Electrical stimulation accelerates and increases expression of BDNF and trkB mRNA in regenerating rat femoral motoneurons. Eur J Neurosci 2000;12:4381–90.

[80] Al-Majed AA, Tam SL, Gordon T. Electrical stimulation accelerates and enhances expression of regeneration-associated genes in regenerating rat femoral motoneurons. Cell Mol Neurobiol 2004;24:379–402.

[81] Anderson CR, Morris RL, Boeh SD, et al. Effects of iontophoresis current magnitude and duration on dexamethasone deposition and localized drug retention. Phys Ther 2003;83: 161–70.

[82] Cagnie B, Vinck E, Rimbaut S, et al. Phonophoresis versus topical application of ketoprofen: comparison between tissue and plasma levels. Phys Ther 2003;83:707–12.

**ELSEVIER
SAUNDERS**

Clin Podiatr Med Surg
23 (2006) 667–672

CLINICS IN
PODIATRIC
MEDICINE AND
SURGERY

Index

Note: Page numbers of article titles are in **boldface** type.

Moving?

Make sure your subscription moves with you!

To notify us of your new address, find your **Clinics Account Number** (located on your mailing label above your name), and contact customer service at:

E-mail: elspcs@elsevier.com

800-654-2452 (subscribers in the U.S. & Canada)
407-345-4000 (subscribers outside of the U.S. & Canada)

Fax number: 407-363-9661

Elsevier Periodicals Customer Service
6277 Sea Harbor Drive
Orlando, FL 32887-4800

*To ensure uninterrupted delivery of your subscription, please notify us at least 4 weeks in advance of move.